Creating a Life
The Memoir of a Writer and Mom in the Making

by Corbin Lewars

CATALYST BOOK PRESS
Livermore, California

Published by Catalyst Book Press
Livermore, California

Copyright © 2010 by Corbin Lewars
Cover Design: Kathy McInnis

Summary: Rape-survivor Corbin Lewars recounts how she reclaimed control of her body—and her life—by becoming a writer and giving birth at home.

Catalyst Book Press would like to thank Tania Pryputniewicz and Lora Parker for their help copy-editing the book.

ISBN 978-0-9802081-5-3
Library of Congress Control Number: 2009931781
January 2010
Printed in the United States of America

To order additional copies of the book, contact Catalyst Book Press
www.catalystbookpress.com
info@catalystbookpress.com
925-606-5992

For Debby
with love

Table of Contents

Introduction
Phyllis Klaus, MFT, LMSW

In her book, *Creating a Life*, Corbin Lewars has been willing to openly face her feelings, reveal her pain, and express her truth. Her story, although uniquely her own, could be a template for others, since 1 out of 4 or 5 girls, and 1 out of 5 or 6 boys, have suffered from childhood sexual abuse. The majority of perpetrators are known to the child and are in some type of power relationship, either physically or emotionally, over the child—such as a family member, an authority figure, or even a peer. The child in most cases has no understanding of the abuse, no knowledge of what is happening, no skills to stop it and no power to give voice to it.

The memories of physical pain and the feelings of confusion, fear, and shame often go underground, or in some way are repressed from conscious awareness. However, the effects of abuse can reverberate throughout one's life, and later affect a person's sense of self, her choices, her relationships, and her sexuality. These effects can especially be activated when she wants to conceive and birth a child.

The efforts to keep at bay the painful feelings and memories are exhausting. The abuse survivor unconsciously works hard to avoid any emotion or reminder of the past trauma and, when events occur that trigger some aspect of an abuse experience, the woman can have a physical response, such as nausea, terror, disorientation. She may do anything to avoid these reactions.

Some women become overachievers; some avoid any emotional connection to their bodies or true sexuality. Others are fearful of being noticed, or speaking up, or asking for what they want. Others pursue a goal with intensity without recognizing their desperation.

Corbin Lewars wanted to have a baby more than anything else. Following this goal, and in other circumstances in her life, she began experiencing some unexpected and highly distressing reactions; she sought therapy to understand them and began making connections to the rapes she suffered as a child. By giving voice and reality to these emotions, they became manageable and she could start to resolve them.

In Corbin Lewars' book, *Creating a Life*, we take a profound step into her inner world. It is an autobiographical window into her soul, her searingly honest voice, into how she faced her worst demons, how they affected her, how she dealt with them, and how she found her voice could give hope and permission to others to take such a risk.

As we step into her world, she writes so openly that she gives the reader an opportunity to test out one's own honesty. Could we ask for what we want? Could we discuss our bodily functions? Could we make personal choices different from our closest friends or relatives even if they protested or did not understand?

Birthing one's baby is so deep, so personal, yet so culturally conditioned that only by the good grace of living in a community that supports midwives, birth centers, or home births could Lewars create the scenario she wanted. We follow her "independent" way of thinking and being, her willingness to check out and research all possibilities, and finally, through psychotherapy, how she learned to trust her gut, her intuition, to listen to her feelings, to go into them, to not avoid them, and in doing so, to learn even more strongly to trust herself.

Each chapter opens another door into her inner world, juxtaposed to real events and choices in her outer world. We learn about her incredibly sweet, kind, "emotionally present" husband, who creates an environment of safety. Any partner of a survivor of abuse could learn from his intuitive ability how to respond to one's partner, how to check with her where she is at emotionally, her level of comfort, and how to remain steadfast without overtaking, how to give her the space to make choices that feel right to her; in other words, to somehow realize how important her ability to have control is without taking offense or judging her.

Her circle of friends provides a comforting foil against which she can learn to ask for what she wants. Each step toward trying out her voice, a voice she never had as a child, becomes healing for her.

We travel her journey of loss of a baby through miscarriage and her risk-taking in career changes.

Corbin has an amazing ability to know that she must heal her abuse traumas before the baby comes because she wants to be the mother to her child and not have the child hold her pain or be the comforter for her. In other words, she knows how easy it would be to use the child to fulfill something in herself and she does not want to do this, so she works hard in therapy to not only heal the past but to separate the past from the present. She develops mantras to repeat during labor—such as "that was then, this is now" to reclaim her power.

The baby's birth at home becomes the ultimate choice of growing through the pain. Her clarity regarding how she researched all the possibilities for birth and made her decision will be immensely informative, realistic, and inspiring to couples planning the birth of their babies—as well as for care providers, especially in this era of unusually high percentage of interventions for birth. Whatever choices they might make, reading about her thoughts, feelings, and information about modern birth practices will be extremely helpful.

More importantly, with her choices of birth attendants, doula, and other support, she created an atmosphere that allowed her the freedom to do what she needed to do to birth her baby. By having no drugs or procedure laden interventions and stepping into her labor with confidence, all her own labor and birth hormones were working in full force. Her body worked the way nature intended through the pain.

You come away from *Creating a Life* relieved, joyful, and stronger—reminded of the human potential to grow and to heal. When asked by her therapist to enumerate all the negative ways the abuse affected her life, she gave a long list, and then was asked for all the positive ways she was affected. She could not think of any—except "opportunity—to have my own voice."

Phyllis Klaus MFT, LMSW is a perinatal psychotherapist, researcher, and co-author of several books including: *Bonding, Your Amazing Newborn, The Doula Book*, and *When Survivors Give Birth: Understanding and Healing the Effects of Child Sexual Abuse on Childbearing Women.*

I
Ringing Clock

Ringing Clock

"I WANT A BABY."

"I know you do."

"So, when do you think we can have one?"

"When I feel ready."

"When will that be?"

"I don't know, but asking me every day isn't going to change things. I need time to think about it; it's a big decision."

"You're right, sorry. I shouldn't rush you. It's important that we're both ready, that we both really want it."

Five minutes later: "Are you ready now?"

And so go the weekly dead-end conversations between my husband Jason and me. Every atom, neuron, and cell in my body is itching to procreate. I see strollers and I cry. I see a onesie or a bootie, and my heart aches. It's all I can do not to mug every woman I see carrying a baby. To say my biological clock is ticking would be the understatement of the year.

Unfortunately, Jason does not share my desire to join together and make a small person. "Can't you just watch Nina's baby when she has it?" he asks. As if any baby will do.

"It's not the same," I whine. "I want my *own* baby."

"Oh." He turns on the television to watch the basketball game, leaving me no other choice but to call Nina.

"How big is it now?" I ask. I settle on to the couch with my wine and pull a chenille throw over me.

"About as big as a football. Is that wine you're slurping? How dare you!" Nina scolds.

I forget that pregnancy has heightened all of her senses, especially when it comes to hearing or smelling things she can no longer have. She sighs on the other end of the phone and I imagine her propping pillows around her enormous belly, striving for the impossible—comfort.

"Sorry. If you were here, I would let you smell it. It's merlot."

"That doesn't work anymore. God, I miss wine. And beer. And the occasional cigarette. And sex. And being able to sleep. And walking. And…"

"But you're going to have a baby!" I interrupt.

"I know and I'm sure it will be worth it, but right now I'd kill for a glass of wine. Nothing beats a glass of red on a cold, damp night. Enjoy it now, because once you're knocked up…."

"I'm starting to think that will never happen."

"He's still not ready? What's he waiting for?"

"I don't know," I sulk. "He claims he enjoys his freedom too much. That he likes going out to see bands, sleeping in late, traveling. But we never travel, so I called bullshit on that one."

"I told you, men are never ready. Just poke a hole in your cervical cap and say it was a miracle. Immaculate conception, or the twenty-first century version of that."

"Really? You think that would work? No, no, no. I can't do that. He'll change his mind soon, I know he will. So tell me about the kicks again. What's it feel like?"

It's conversations like these that have earned me the name "baby-buzzard" from my sister Stacy. She claims that I stalk pregnant women and befriend them only because they're pregnant. She says I'm obsessed. Maybe I am, but I'll never admit that to her.

I earned the name shortly after my friend Lydia became pregnant. In my defense, I was friends with Lydia before she was pregnant, but Stacy ignored that fact. She rolled her eyes when I talked about Lydia's pregnancy and scoffed at me when I said I couldn't wait to attend the birth. When Lydia found one too many hypodermic needles on the ground in front of her Capitol Hill apartment, she moved to the east side. When I continued to visit her in that cultural wasteland, my sister said, "That's it, baby-buzzard, you need help."

I don't really blame Lydia for moving to the land of ranch homes and back yards. I loved the old wood floors and stucco ceilings of her old apartment, but her baby had to sleep in the closet. And the main attraction to living on Capitol Hill is being near fun bars and in the center of Seattle's gay community, both of which Lydia's baby couldn't care less about. So she's traded in the needles and nightlife for a fenced backyard and a dog. And I've cemented my baby buzzard status by actually visiting her there.

Although older than me, Stacy obviously doesn't hear her own biological clock ticking. Maybe she doesn't even have a clock. Maybe I have hers and that's why mine sounds so loud.

She seems content to continue working like a dog and then spending the money she earns eating and drinking in Seattle's finest restaurants. "Over one hundred thousand dollars flushed down the sewers," Stacy's boyfriend lamented after doing their taxes this year. "What do we have to show for it? Nothing."

Staying out late and spending all of my money on frivolities lost my interest a while ago. Last year I went to Bali with Stacy and, within an hour of being there, told her, "This place looks a lot like Hawaii, except it took us twenty hours to get here. A beach is a beach. It would be a lot cooler if we had kids to play with."

She shook her head in disappointment. "You're so jaded, baby buzzard. Stop being a downer and pass me the sun block."

I know that Jason isn't ready, so at first I keep the desire to have a baby to myself. I try to curb my yearnings by staying busy. I learn that the university I work for will pay for my Master's Degree, so I apply to the Education Department. I'm accepted and throw myself into the course work. About half way through the program, the baby stalking returns, so I convince Jason we need to remodel our house.

I spend every weekend either writing papers about the multiple intelligences and literacies that homeless women possess or putting up insulation, smoothing drywall, and installing junction boxes. It takes walking into the kitchen to find rain dripping through our makeshift blue tarp roof right onto my keyboard for me to realize I'm living a crazy life. The computer won't turn on, I have several papers due in the morning, and our tiny kitchen is the only non-construction place to work, cook, and eat. I'm busy to the point of exhaustion, my house is in shambles, yet I'm still restless.

When I share all of this with my friend Jennifer, she says, "What if...." She pauses and I can tell she's choosing her words very carefully. "What if having a baby isn't the solution either?"

"What!? Of course it is. I've been pining for one for years. That's the project I really want, but until Jason's ready, I'm making do with a remodel."

"I'm just wondering if you're running away from something or running towards something? Maybe you could take a break from all of the projects and take some time to think about what's really driving your dissatisfaction."

Jennifer's words strike a nerve and I don't like it. I haven't felt satisfied in years, so I constantly search for the next project that will fill the gap I feel in my life. But I don't think I'm avoiding anything; I'm just restless.

"I don't want to take a break, I want a baby. I'm sure that's the thing that will satisfy me," I say defensively.

She raises her eyebrows at me, letting me know she doesn't believe me, but when I start to argue my case more, she lifts her hands in a plea of surrender. "It's your life, you know best. I'm just worried about you, that's all. You've gone into debt and are running yourself ragged..."

"Don't worry, I'm fine," I say.

I feel irritated with Jennifer and want to prove her wrong. But maybe there's some truth to what she says. Graduate school and the remodel keep me busy, yet I still feel dissatisfied. Even worse, it pushes any notions of procreating to the furthest recesses of Jason's brain. He doesn't think about having a baby while drywalling, he thinks about drywall. And now that we finally have a roof over our heads and drywall on the walls, he wants to relax, leaving me in no-baby purgatory for all that much longer. Unless I follow Nina's advice and poke a hole in my cervical cap. Sure, Jason will be pissed at first, but he'll get over it once he sees our beautiful baby. Right?

POKING A HOLE IN MY CERVICAL CAP may get me pregnant, but it could also get me divorced. I'll have to think of something else. Maybe I can find a better job. An interesting, creative, writing job that I can do from home. Who am I kidding? Those jobs don't exist. I'll be stuck at Fruitloop U forever.

It's not that Fruitloop U is such an awful place to work, it's just not where I want to work. The faculty love to "discuss" things, but rarely want to do anything about what we discuss. I spend my days in meetings where even the "discussions" are vague, esoteric, and full of sentences beginning with "Epistemologically speaking…" Is that even a word? If it's not, someone better let the faculty at Fruitloop U know.

I'm not much for discussing pedagogies, theories, or comparing epistemological notes. I know it's strange, but I think work is a place where you should get things done. I really blew them away with that concept when they first hired me. After my initial tour and introductions to everyone in my department, I said, "All right, what should I do now?" Hank, my tour guide and the person responsible for training me, said, "Why don't you take some time to get the feel of the department?" Apparently, he thought that should take two weeks.

I try to remain motivated and to create my own projects, but it's hard not to view my efforts as futile. I'm the Student Liaison for a small graduate program. Not only are there not that many students to "liaison" for, but combine that with the faculty's indifference to the students' ideas, and I end up having a lot of free time on my hands.

I'm the complaints department at best, a trash can at worst. I provide a place for the faculty to send disgruntled students, but once they come to me, no one wants to hear from them again. No one cares what I do all day; they just want me to be here. I spend most of my time talking to friends on the phone or visiting with colleagues at work. When I'm not socializing, I'm busy with my own projects. How do you think I earned a Master's Degree and remodeled a house while working full time?

I'm probably just being passive aggressive and hoping they fire me for being a slacker. These days I'm hardly even there. I spend every morning, like this morning, dinking around my house and daydreaming over coffee. I claim I'm trying to avoid traffic, but really I'm avoiding work.

Once the gazing is over and my errands are complete, I finally decide to grace Fruitloop U with my presence. I pop the White Stripes into the CD player as a way to enhance my last few minutes of freedom. I sing along to "Seven Nation Army" as I drive down Fifteenth Avenue. "…talking to myself a lot because I can't forget…." It's nearly ten thirty when I pull into the parking lot, but I stay in the car to hear "The Hardest Button to Button."

A colleague says the education department has free pastries, derailing work all the longer. I shove two in my mouth and take a third for the road before finally arriving at my office. The red light on my phone is blinking accusingly at me. I flop down in my chair and listen half-heartedly as I check my emails.

"Corbin, I hope you get this message soon. It's Tony and Nina's in labor. Call me at home."

Next message. "Corbin, it's Tony again. Her contractions are coming really quickly. We're at the hospital. Call me …."

Message from student asking about fall registration. Classes started a month ago, so I skip the message.

Message from my boss, which I also skip.

"Corbin, where the hell are you! She's almost fully dilated. Get your ass up here! We're in room 302."

After this message, I grab my coat, write "Out to lunch, be back soon" on my door, and drive to the hospital.

"Don't have the baby without me," I say whenever I have to stop at a light. I curse the pouring rain, which prohibits me and all of the other cars from speeding. I accidentally spray a bunch of pedestrians with the puddle I tear through as I take a right on Denny. Remembering Lydia's birth, I calm down a bit and take my foot off the accelerator.

I received several frantic phone calls from Lydia's partner as well and when I got there, Lydia wasn't even considered to be in "active labor" yet. At least that's what the nurses said. She sure seemed active to me. She was screaming and crying and swearing up a storm. Every time the nurse entered the room, Lydia screamed, "I need drugs!" When the nurse recommended a hot tub or changing positions, Lydia screamed, "I've tried all of that shit! Give me drugs!" Finally, the nurses conceded and ordered an epidural for Lydia, but it didn't seem to help. She continued to scream for more drugs and soon was on a first name basis with the anesthesiologist. Whenever Dan, the man with the drugs, left the room, Lydia screamed. When a contraction came, Lydia screamed. When her partner told her it was going to be all right or tried to touch her in any way, she yelled profanities at him. After about eight or ten hours of this, her baby was finally born. Then Lydia hemorrhaged and blood came pouring out of her at a very unnatural rate. As the doctor jumped up and down on her abdomen, I vowed to adopt. I also contemplated revoking my baby buzzard status.

But as soon as Nina became pregnant, I was enraptured. After barraging her with ten thousand questions and calling her after every midwife appointment, she said the magical words, "You can be there if you want."

I told Nina about Lydia's birth, but she claims she doesn't want any drugs. She explicitly told her midwives, "No drugs, don't even offer them to me." That sounds nice, in theory, but I don't think it's possible. Unless you're Super Woman or something.

NINA IS SUPER WOMAN. No, she's a lion. A bear? A…. Well, at the moment she's a naked pregnant woman squatting on the ground.

After ripping the IV out of her arm and stripping all of her clothes off, she bats the nurse away. Her partner Tony is the only one who seems to be able to interpret her grunts and mumbles. They're in their own world. Nurses come and go while Nina paces back and forth, emitting the occasional howl. She's gone inside of herself and is completely oblivious to her surroundings and the people in the room. She could be in the woods for all she cares. Occasionally, she'll squeeze Tony's hand or grab on to his shoulders when she lets out a groan, but mostly she takes care of herself. I can't help feeling as if I'm Jane Goodall, studying the behavior of a wild animal.

The nurses chat about the latte they wish they had as they run washcloths under cold water. They smile as they offer Nina yoga balls and don't even flinch when she growls at them. They merely continue rinsing and chatting as if listening to a naked woman howl is a normal everyday occasion.

Although I don't spend a lot of time with naked, howling women, there is something natural about this situation. When I focus on Nina, I forget we're in a hospital. Besides the IV to regulate her high blood pressure, no other foreign substances or steel objects have been used to aid her progress. She drinks water occasionally, but otherwise relies on her body and her mind to get her through each contraction.

It's such a contrast to Lydia's birth. Lydia remained in bed, on her back, the entire time. Next to her was a tray of surgical instruments, several machines beeping and hissing intermittently, and three or four nurses constantly adjusting the tubes and IVs coming out of her. I never once forgot I was in a hospital.

Rather than feeling comforted by the copious staff and machinery, I felt agitated. I paced back and forth and even had to leave the room several times. I kept flashing back to the last time I was in a hospital. At a routine pelvic exam, my doctor said I might have dysplasia and suggested I come back in a few weeks for a biopsy. She didn't explain what a biopsy was or what dysplasia was; all she said was she found some abnormal blood cells on my cervix and it could lead to cervical cancer. She told me not to worry (which of course I did) and sent me home.

When I went in for the biopsy, I found all the nurses at the hospital shivering and rubbing their hands together. The central heating wasn't working, so everyone was making do with a space heater and lots of layers. That is, everyone but me. All I was wearing was a flimsy paper gown. It didn't help that the nurses continually commented on how cold the room was and blocked all the heat from the space heater, which was nowhere near me, the only naked person.

The doctor asked me to relax as she placed my legs in stirrups. I had understood that a biopsy was a routine procedure where the doctor would take a sampling of my cervix to be further examined in a lab. Instead, it felt like she was removing my uterus. She took six sections of my cervix and each time I felt excruciating cramping. I cried, shivered, and worried that I would defecate all over the examining table, yet no one consoled me. They just looked at me and kept saying, "It sure is cold in here." When it was finally over, I tried to sit up, but when I glanced down between my legs, I saw blood all over the examining table. For fear of fainting, I laid back down.

I couldn't help but project my fear and confusion from the biopsy onto Lydia's labor. It felt as if she was being held captive in her bed and I couldn't tolerate just standing around watching. I wanted to help, but didn't know how. My offers of cool washcloths and massages didn't stop her from screaming and I didn't know how else to relieve her pain. It didn't look like any of the other people in the room were helping much either.

Nina doesn't appear to be in pain, nor does she seem to need any help. Sure, she's howling and groaning, but it seems to be aiding her labor, whereas Lydia's screams seemed to come from a place of fear. I can see that Nina is in control and is confident in her body, allowing me to feel relaxed in a way I never felt during Lydia's birth.

Drugs are never mentioned and I can only imagine what Nina's response would be if they were, seeing as she looks like she might bite the nurse's arm off if she rolls that damn yoga ball in front of her again. She doesn't want a ball, hot tub, or even a cool washcloth; she just wants to be left alone.

Nina's howls turn to grunts and she begins squatting while grabbing Tony's shoulders. The nurses exchange looks. One of them says, "Based on that grunt you just let out, I'd say you're in the pushing stage. Want to hold onto this bar and squat?"

Nina completely ignores the nurse and resumes her frantic pacing and grunting. The nurse finally convinces her she's due for an exam and that it will not be conducted while she's lying on the floor. Three nurses hoist Nina on to the bed, and sure enough, she's fully dilated.

As soon as the nurses release Nina, she resumes her pacing. Blood trickles down her leg as she crosses the room. I'm obviously the only one disturbed by this, because no one else says or does anything about the red pool on the floor. They don't even bother to clean it up. One of the nurses throws a cloth on the ground and Nina continues pacing and squatting over it.

As soon as Nina screams, "Ow, it burns!", the nurses lose their pleasant, agreeable demeanors and get down to business. They pull and tug on the bed, raise the back, drop the front, and change the sheets. They fasten a bar over the bed and place a stool at the foot.

"Listen to me, Nina," one of them says as she holds Nina's face in her hands and looks her square in the eye. "That means the baby's head is crowning, which means it's coming soon. I need you to be still so we can help you. You can hold on to this bar or…" Nina shakes her head violently. "All right," the nurse continues. She grabs Tony and Nina and walks them over to the bed while another nurse removes the bar. Two nurses hoist Nina up on the bed and place Tony in front of her. Nina grabs hold of his shoulders, stands up on the bed, and squats and groans. Before she can get off the bed again, two nurses grab her shoulders, recline her body, and tell her to rest. They scurry Tony around to Nina's side, and then one of them places herself at the foot of Nina's bed. They tell me to hold Nina's leg up to her chest when the contractions come.

Once everyone is in position and understands their duties, the nurses place all of their attention back on Nina. They obviously watch a lot of *Law and Order*, because they have the good cop, bad cop thing down perfectly. The tough one holds Nina's face while talking firmly to her, while the nice ones coo and offer her ice chips. I think the woman at the foot of the bed is the midwife. It's hard to tell because they are all dressed the same, bustle around in the same manner, and use the same language and tone with one another. There is no apparent hierarchy and none of the "Yes Doctor, No Doctor, whatever you say, Doctor," that I usually hear in hospitals.

"OWWWWWW!" Nina screams.

All of the nurses, and the midwife, cheer her on. "That was beautiful. A few more of those and you'll get to hold your baby. You're doing great, just great. Rest until you feel the next contraction."

"Owwwww!" she screams again. Tony's face is contorted and I can't tell if it's due to concern over Nina or pain from the death-hold she has on his hand. I smile at him and he smiles weakly back.

"It burns!" she screams again.

"Good, good," they say. The midwife asks us if we want to see the baby's head. Tony looks at Nina and his now white hand, which Nina is squeezing too hard, and shakes his head. I say, "Sure," and move closer to the midwife. I see a mass of black slimy stuff creep out of Nina's vagina as she screams "Owww!" again. It slides back in as soon as she leans back.

"That's the baby?" I ask, feeling slightly dizzy.

"Yup. Another one just like that, Nina. Tuck your chin to your chest and give it all you got."

Several, maybe a hundred, pushes later—who knows, time has become surreal—the head finally comes out and stays out. We hear a big "sluuuurp" and a red, gooey, screaming thing slides into the midwife's hands. A lot more red and yellow stuff pours out of Nina's vagina and into a bag that is placed at the foot of the bed. Well, some of it makes it into the bag and some of it pours all over the floor. I try to focus on the baby and not the blood, but I can't keep my eyes off of it. *How can so much stuff come out of such a tiny woman? Is that supposed to happen or is she hemorrhaging like Lydia did? Why isn't anyone trying to stop it?*

As steadily as I can, I walk away from the foot of the bed and towards Nina's head. I'm sure I'll faint if I keep looking at all of that blood. I'm usually not a squeamish person. Bugs, snakes, even blood and guts in movies don't faze me. And even though I know that the midwife will help Nina if she's in danger, I still fear for her. I can't shake the feeling that she's being hurt.

"She's beautiful, just beautiful," they all say. The midwife places the baby onto Nina's chest. The nurse pulls the blankets up over mother and baby, and smiles at both of them. "Good work, Mom." Nina is still bleeding, but not at an alarming rate, so I tell myself everything is under control. I can relax.

After a few minutes of baby appreciation, the midwife looks at Tony and says, "Ready to cut the cord, Dad?" He nods and listens intently to the instructions. "Wait until it stops pulsing," she says. "Yes, right there would be good. All right, go ahead."

Snip and splat! Blood splatters all the way across the room and sprays my arm and shirt. "Uh, is this hygienic?" I ask. I look around for a tissue or washcloth to clean myself with, but no one pays me any attention. The nurse asks Nina if she wants to keep the placenta. Nina nods, and I watch as more blood and mucus are passed back and forth while the nurses look for a bag to place the placenta in. Before they put it away, they make sure we all have a good look at it to see how healthy and red it is.

"And see, there's the tree of life," the midwife marvels as she points to a bunch of veiny looking things. I don't see a tree, but am not about to ask for clarification.

The nurses continue to bustle around and clean up, before slowly trickling out of the room. They smile at Nina, who is gazing adoringly at her baby, and tell her she was amazing. They dim the lights as they go and I start to feel like an intruder. I give the new family a hug and say goodbye as well.

I have to sit in my car for a few minutes to gather myself. What an amazing experience. It was so calm and natural. Sure, I could have done without some of the blood and goo, but Nina's strength was impressive. I can't believe how focused and relaxed she was throughout the whole labor. She knew what she needed and never asked for drugs. I didn't think it was possible.

I glance at the clock and panic. It's nearly five o'clock and I've done nothing for work all day! I race down Capitol Hill back to work.

"Hey, you missed the meeting about ....." a colleague starts as soon as I enter the door of my department. "Are you all right? You look a little frazzled. Where have you been?"

"Nina's birth. She was amazing. She was like a bear, so feral, so primal, you would never have believed it. She was completely in control of her body. She's incredible..." I babble.

"Is that blood on your shirt?" he asks as he takes a step back.

I glance down and see the dark red smear. "Yeah, I guess it is. Gross." I try to rub it with my hand, but it's dry. I look up and continue my ramblings, but stop when I notice he's gone. In fact, he's running down the hallway.

"I'M IN LOVE WITH NINA'S BABY," I tell Jason over dinner. "Do you think she'd let me have her?"

"People don't give their babies as presents. You're a little crazy about this, you know?"

"No, I'm not. I just figured that way I wouldn't have to wait for you to be ready. I wouldn't have to go through labor or pregnancy, I could just have a beautiful baby girl now! It would be perfect."

"It's not going to happen. It's her baby, not yours. All right?"

I tell myself Jason is wrong, he doesn't know Nina as well as I do. She wasn't even trying to get pregnant, it just happened to her, so I'm sure it could happen again. She can have her next baby and give me Estelle. I smile at the memory of her curled up in my arms, sound asleep with a smile on her face. I think she loves me.

"Aren't you going to get in trouble at work? I mean, you've hardly been there since Estelle was born," he asks.

"We're rarely busy and no one seems to care that I'm gone. There's a new rumor going around that our department might be shut down, so everyone is more concerned about that than my whereabouts."

"You could be laid off?"

I shrug. "Worse things could happen. At least then I'd get unemployment."

"You find the strangest jobs. Have you ever worked somewhere normal? With normal people and normal hours?"

"I worked for you," I laugh. "Was that normal?"

"No! That place was a freak show." Jason and I worked together in a coffee shop in Bellingham, the town Jason was born and raised in. Well, I should clarify. Jason worked: he was a manager. I spent most of my time eating, talking to my coworkers, and slipping over to the bar up the street whenever possible. Sounds like how we spend our days now.

Although Jason isn't thrilled about his job at Ivey, he still works really hard all day long. He mounts photographs to plexiglass, hangs enormous displays in store windows, or otherwise does what is expected of him. He knows the job is beneath him and doesn't plan on making a career of it, yet he works steadily while he's there. I, on the other hand, still spend the majority of my time at work socializing. At least I don't go to bars anymore. I could view that as progress, but really it's just because there aren't any cool bars near Fruitloop U.

"Remember when I gave you that awful review? I was so scared you were going to be pissed and instead you hugged me and pranced out the door." Jason shakes his head at the memory.

"As soon as you said, 'You seem to get along with the other employees,' I conveniently forgot the rest of the review where you asked me to stop swearing in front of the customers, stop having half hour phone conversations with my boyfriend, and stop turning my ten minute breaks into hour long drinking sprees. That was a fun job."

"For you."

Jason starts to clear our dishes while I stare out the window and reminisce about our coffee shop days. Jason was the manager everyone loved to work with. He knew almost everyone in town, having lived there his whole life, and was the softie who never got angry with anyone. I warned him that he was going to get taken advantage of, but he said his niceness was his strategy to get people to do what he wanted. And it worked, for the most part.

The sun peeks through the clouds and fills our kitchen with light. It's right in my eyes, but I don't move. It's such a treat to feel its warmth after a couple weeks of rain. I would enjoy fall so much more, with all of its glorious colors and crisp air, if it wasn't a constant reminder of what's ahead: winter.

On his way to the sink, Jason pauses. "Do you think you could clean up your language for the baby?"

"Nina's baby? She can barely open her eyes much less understand what asshole means."

"No, our baby. I don't want its first word to be 'fuck.' Can you work on the potty mouth?"

"We're going to have a baby!" I squeal. That's all I hear him say. The foul mouth lecture is tuned out.

"Yeah, I've been thinking about it. But did you hear what I said about the swearing? Maybe start practicing now so by the time…"

I grab his hand and pull him up the stairs to our bedroom. Screw the dirty dishes and lectures, I want a baby!

II
Conception

Conception

"YOU'RE JUST USING ME for my sperm," Jason says.

I'm about to protest, but realize he might be right. I have been a little demanding lately. But you would think any guy would be thrilled to have their wife want sex every day. Especially a wife they've been with for seven years. Better to have sex with him than fall privy to the "seven-year-itch" and start having sex elsewhere.

As soon as he announced he was ready, I stripped off my clothes. And since then I have been pretty intense about this. Who knew unprotected sex could be so exciting? Not me. I don't think I've ever had it before now. Throughout my late teens and twenties, I was on the birth control pill. I was one of those girls who went on the pill as soon as she even considered having sex. No unexpected pregnancy for me, no way! Then I stayed on it for years and years. In between boyfriends, I would consider going off of it, but the "what if" factor always kept me on it. "What if I meet someone cool?" "What if I get drunk and get together with someone?" What I never considered were the following questions: what if I got a backbone and told the guy to put a condom on? what if I said "no?" I didn't know how to stand up for myself, so I protected myself in the only way I knew how—by making sure I didn't get pregnant.

I never liked taking the pill or the effect it had on my emotions every month, so once Jason and I had been together for a few years, I went off of it. We quickly learned that condoms sucked (which isn't to say I should not have used them before!) so I opted for the cervical cap. Mixed with spermicidal gel and the occasional condom on top, just to be sure.

But now I'm liberated! I throw the spermicide away and toss the condoms with them. It's almost as good as the sex we had when we first met. Even better in some ways, because I might get a baby out of it!

"I mean, you don't even care how we do it, you just want to do it. At first it was fun, but now it's kinda freaky." Jason buttons his jeans and pulls his shirt over his head without looking at me. A sure sign he's pissed.

I know he's right and even though we've been having a lot of sex, it hasn't necessarily been good sex. I don't want to mess around with foreplay, I just want to make a baby. I become tense and rigid whenever he caresses my body or strokes my clitoris. I don't care about being turned on, sometimes it even makes me feel uncomfortable to be touched. I just want to have his sperm inside of me. But I don't tell him this, for fear of hurting his feelings. Plus, he might cut me off from sex if he knew what I was really thinking.

"Well, it's just that I waited for so long for you to be ready and now that you finally are, I'm excited. I want it to happen. In fact, I can't believe it hasn't happened already. We've really been going at it."

"It's only been a few months, maybe…"

"Four months, it's been four long months."

"That's not that long. Maybe you need to relax and not get so fixated on it."

"I hate it when people tell me to relax."

"I know you do, but you should listen to them sometimes." He walks downstairs to make coffee.

I stay in bed to give myself time to think. If I freak Jason out too much, there will be no baby. And no unprotected sex. Although I hate the "relax" word, I'll try. I'll try to forget about my burning desire to procreate. I'll try to stop thinking every little stomach quiver is a baby being conceived. I'll try to stop crying every month when I get my period. I'll try to forget all of this and act like a normal person.

Yeah, right. That will never work. I need another project. I need something I can see the beginning and end of. Something I can control. Something I can be in charge of. But what? I'm out of ideas. And the remodeling and grad school frenzy didn't help matters. Sure, I was busy, but I still wasn't satisfied.

I guess I could throw myself into my work like every other person my age in Seattle. Ha! That's funny. They'd fall over at Fruitloop U if I ever showed my face before ten o'clock. Speaking of—I glance at the clock—I better get ready.

It's nearly ten thirty by the time I arrive at work. I walk into our department and groan when I see Mark waiting for me. It's not that Mark is a horrible person; he's kind of funny and very nice. It's just that he, like many students before him, wants to know what exactly he is receiving for his fifty thousand dollar tuition.

The last time we met he wanted to know what jobs he'll be eligible for when he graduates. The unfortunate answer is, "I have no idea." Our department has an alarmingly large amount of unemployed graduates. I didn't tell this to Mark; instead I distracted him by telling him there were free cookies in the Psych department. I wonder if that will work today.

"Hey, Mark. Are you here to see me?"

"No, I'm waiting to see my advisor."

"Cool," I say with a bit too much enthusiasm. I can hardly contain my relief as I open my office door. I put my bag down and check my messages. Amongst the many "I missed class, so could you…" and "Professor Z hasn't returned my phone calls in over three weeks, is he out of town?" phone calls, there is one interesting one.

"Corbin, this is Karen, remember me? I'm an alumnus from a few years back and met you in the office a few times. Anyway, I'm embarking on a really exciting project that you may be interested in. Check your emails. I wrote you all about it."

At Fruitloop U, you never know what an "exciting project" could be. For months, a group of students have been trying to convince me to join them in building a straw-bale house. I'm not too excited about that project, seeing as it's winter and I can't imagine how warm or dry straw is, but I am curious about Karen's idea.

Her email begins with a description of a small newspaper called *Women of Seattle*. The paper is for sale and Karen is hoping to gather a collective of women who would like to buy it with her. I'm about to delete the email, knowing that I don't have any money to contribute to the cause, but maybe I could offer some help. I used to work in publishing and loved the fast pace, the deadlines, the continuous cycle of newness that comes with always having another issue to put out. It would be better than sitting in this office all day. This could be just the thing I'm looking for. A creative job and something to take my mind off my baby obsession.

I call her and hear about her big dreams of turning this small, local newspaper into a beautiful publication that every woman in Seattle will read. *Women of Seattle* is a trade publication, geared for women entrepreneurs and business owners. Karen wants to expand the audience and expand the content to include health, relationships, law advice, and inspirational stories about women giving up on lucrative but unfulfilling careers to embark on projects they feel more passionate about.

I get so carried away in her dream that I never hear the specifics of what is going to happen. She says she needs help soon, sounds enthusiastic when I explain my background in publishing, and says she knows how good I am with people from my work at Fruitloop U. I have to laugh at that.

I'm not sure what kind of help she will need exactly, but she says I can work from home, have a flexible schedule, and she'll try to come up with a base salary for me. The working from home and creative element sells me. It's my dream job. The one I thought didn't exist. No more being bored! No more feeling underutilized! No more two hour meetings about pedagogies! I'm free at last!

I tell Karen it sounds perfect and we set a time to meet the following week. I bounce around in my seat and crank the stereo on the drive home from work. I sing along with KEXP at the top of my lungs. At a commercial break, my enthusiasm wanes and Jennifer's words come to mind. "Are you running toward something or away from something?" Is working with Karen another distraction?

The more I recall the conversation with Karen, the more I'm convinced working for her isn't just a diversion, it's a move in the right direction. If there's any truth to Jennifer's words, that I'm avoiding something or missing something in my life and hoping a baby will solve my problems, then I need to fix that now. I can't expect a baby to totally fulfill me; I need to do that for myself. And I need to do it before I have a baby. The baby will need *me*. I can't need it.

I think part of my baby craze is looking for an escape from Fruitloop U. But I don't need to be pregnant in order to quit. I could quit now!

By the time I pull into my driveway, I know working for Karen is the right thing. Karen is offering an opportunity I've dreamt about for years. Sure, it involves risk, but if I pass it up, I'll regret it. It's not only an opportunity to have a creative job that will challenge me, but also the chance to prove to myself that I have the courage to go for what I want. This is definitely running towards something, not running away.

As soon as I walk into our house, I announce to Jason that I'm quitting.

"Sure you are," he says.

"No, really, I've found the perfect job." I tell him all about Karen and *Women of Seattle*.

"I know you're sick of Fruitloop U, but it seems so sudden. Can Karen pay you enough to live on?"

His question bursts my bubble a bit, but I'm determined to make it work. "We didn't sort out all of the details yet, but I can always teach on a contract basis again if I need to."

"I thought you were burned out on teaching."

Damn him for being so practical! I'm trying to go out on a limb here and he's not helping. And how come he's choosing this moment to actually remember what I say? He's right, I am tired of teaching. I started teaching writing on a part time basis as another way to escape Fruitloop U, but I can't say I'm passionate about it. Just because I love writing doesn't mean I love *teaching* writing.

"If I have to teach, I will. But it will be great if Karen can pay me enough to live on, because that's more what I want to do. I love working in publishing and it would be great to be surrounded by women who are actually creating the life they want and are excited about things. It would be so cool to be a part of something positive, something that helps people, something that people can learn from."

I laugh as I realize this is exactly what Fruitloop U claims to be. I'm practically quoting their mission statement. Yet I've never felt as if I'm making a difference there.

"I guess that's what I thought it would be like to work at Fruitloop U," I say.

"Yeah, you were really optimistic when you started there."

I was certain after three sets of interviews, many visits to the campus, and four secret phone calls to Fruitloop U employees I knew through friends of friends, that it was the place for me. And I was wrong. So this time around, I want to try listening to my gut and not my head. My head will weigh pros and cons, become nervous about the unknown salary and job responsibilities, and question the feasibility and longevity of the paper, whereas my gut says, "Who cares about all of that? I'm ready for a change and this sounds like a great opportunity. I want to start making my life be the way I want it to be, not the way I think it should be. Even if it doesn't work out, it will free me from Fruitloop U, which is a step in the right direction."

This time, I'm going with my gut.

"HOW DID IT GO?" Jennifer asks as we walk to our cars.

"Surprisingly well. Barbara was very understanding about my desire to find a more creative job and was so pleased to hear about Karen and her publishing endeavors that she seemed to forget all about me quitting. Overall, it was easier than I expected. There was one caveat that I wasn't prepared for."

"What's that?"

"She wants me to stay on for a couple more months to help things get sorted out for my replacement."

"Oh, what do you think of that?"

"I'm not sure. In a way, the steady paycheck could be nice because I don't have anything else that's solid yet. And I could go see the doctor, while I still have insurance, and…"

"I thought you couldn't wait to get out of here. To be the new Corbin, going for what she wants and not letting fear stand in her way."

I know Jennifer is only teasing me, but I cringe at hearing my words thrown back at me. She's right, I do want to figure out what I need and go for it, rather than settle for the easy but boring path. But a steady paycheck for a few months sure would be nice.

I keep these thoughts to myself when Sonya catches up to us. Word that I quit will be out soon enough. I don't need big-mouth-Sonya spreading the news tonight. I want to have a clear end-date before I tell people I'm leaving.

"What are you guys doing for Valentine's Day?" Sonya asks.

She mostly looks at Jennifer, the single girl.

"I'm going salsa dancing," Jennifer replies.

A long pause follows, so I share my plans as well. "We wanted to go out of town for the three-day weekend, but we're kind of broke, so I had an idea. What if I made a special dinner, bought some champagne, and then lit a bunch of candles in our guest room and we pretended we were in a nice hotel?"

"It could work," Jennifer smiles as Sonya says, "That's lame. What are you trying to do, be romantic?"

"Yeah. Who knows, we may even have hot sex."

I don't even have the words out of my mouth before they both crack up.

"But you're married!" Sonya squeals. "Valentine's Day, romance, and hot sex are for people who are dating, not old married people like you."

"But…" I stop myself from explaining that I've almost killed my sex life with Jason by demanding it all of the time and that for the first time in a while maybe we can create an atmosphere of romance and relaxation instead of getting right down to business. I'm not ready to share the baby secret yet and I also don't feel like defending all "old married couples" who are hoping to spice things up now and then, so all I say is, "You'll see. It's going to be great. Romantic and sexy."

"I hope it is." Jennifer smiles.

Sonya says, "Yeah, yeah," and walks to her car.

Determined to prove Sonya wrong, I start brainstorming a grocery list as I drive home. At a stop light, I rummage through CDs, coffee cups, jackets, something sticky in a bakery bag, and finally find a receipt large enough to write on.

Champagne

Crabcakes, I think I can buy them already made at the fish counter

Risotto

Parmesan cheese

Chicken broth

Onion

Mixed greens for salad

Blue cheese

Pears

Dried cranberries

Sugared pecans, maybe I can sugar them myself. How hard can it be?

I'm so busy thinking about dinner and ingredients that I drive right by the grocery store. I'm nearly home at this point, so decide to run in and change my clothes before I go to the store. I'm surprised to see Jason's Mazda already in the driveway and even more surprised to see him standing over the stove when I walk into the kitchen.

"You're home early. What's up?" I drop my bag on the floor and kick my shoes off. They land in a heap with all of my other shoes. The first thing I always do when I get home is take my shoes off and then wash my face. As if the outside world is dirty and I have to wash its residue off.

"Going to put your pajamas on?" Jason smiles. He knows that's the third thing I like to do when I get home.

"No, I'm gonna run back out to the store. But maybe I could put most of my pjs on and hide them under my coat. And my slippers kind of look like shoes, right?"

"Not really," he laughs. "What do ya have to go to the store for? I've got dinner covered."

"You do?"

"Yeah, it's all set. Here, take this with you while you change." He walks to the stand-up cabinet, pulls out the champagne flutes we stole from the Cloud Room on the night he proposed to me, and pours us both a glass of champagne. "Happy Valentine's Day." We clink glasses, hug and kiss, and then smile at one another as we take our first sip.

"And here's to change," he continues. "Did you tell Barbara today?"

"Yeah, but she wants me to stay on for a few months."

"Why? Once someone quits, they're dead weight."

"Honey, I already was dead weight. Yum, this is good." I take another sip of champagne. "And what are you making? It smells great."

"Fettuccine Alfredo, crabcakes, and salad. The special salad you like with the sugared pecans. They're toasting in the oven right now. It will be ready in about fifteen minutes. Do you want me to slow it down?"

"No, that sounds perfect. I'll go change and then I can help you."

I pass a stack of mail on my way to our room, but ignore it. I don't want to deal with bills or anything obligatory tonight. We're on vacation, after all. With that in mind, I turn the phone ringer off and head upstairs to change. When I get there, I see all of the lights are off and about thirty candles are lit, bathing the guest room in a gorgeous, soft, sensual light. A big bouquet of flowers is perched prominently on the table and soft music is playing. I enter our room and find more of the same. The smell of lilies and aromatherapy candles blends with the rich smell of butter and cream coming from downstairs.

I strip off my clothes, reach for one of Jason's old t-shirts, and pause. No, this calls for something special, something better than an old Radiohead t-shirt. I want to dress for romance. I search around for something sexy, and flinch at my choices of "lingerie." Practical, cotton underwear all of a somewhat nondescript color from too many washings. Instead of a lacy, sexy push up bra I find a couple of stretched out Jockey bras, worn through in spots. And not in a sexy see-through way.

I sigh with the realization that my lingerie is a metaphor for my sex life: practical and a bit worn out. When did this happen and why? I can't remember the last time I actually enjoyed sex for sex's sake, not its baby making qualities. Have I always been this way or is it just because I want a baby so much?

But I don't want to feel that way tonight. I dig a little deeper and find a tight, lacy camisole that I bought for myself years ago. I search for a comparable bottom, but have to settle for my flannel pajama pants. I squeeze into the camisole and force myself to look in the mirror. Not great, but not horrible either. The camisole squishes my breasts into something that sort of resembles cleavage and hugs my waist in a flattering way. Maybe there's hope for romance after all. Even for an old married couple.

Jason gives me a quizzical look when I enter the kitchen. "You look nice. I haven't seen that on you in awhile."

"Thanks and thank you for the flowers. They're amazing." I wrap my arms around his neck and say, "What do you think about postponing dinner for a bit?"

He smiles as I take his hand and lead him upstairs, grabbing the champagne bottle on our way.

IN ORDER TO CELEBRATE MY soon-to-be-freedom as well as my thirty-first birthday, Stacy and I fly to Palm Springs. I always love a trip to somewhere warm and sunny in March, when it's been overcast and rainy in Seattle for months, but I'm not sure right now is the best time for a vacation. I should be spending my time sorting things out with Karen or looking for more work. Stacy convinces me by saying it will be a cheap, short vacation. "You may as well take advantage of getting paid while you're not working now, because it's about to come to an end."

I find a perfectly reasonable hotel for $160 a night. It's near downtown, so we won't need to rent a car, and it has a swimming pool. What else do we need? Stacy has other ideas. A $400 a night room, further away from town, but with a "retro, kitschy" theme. Stacy, being a designer, cares about such things.

I, being barely employed, don't. But she offers to pay for the majority of it, so "retro kitsch" it is.

I immediately see it's not worth $400 a night. It's pretty small, a bit rundown, and the swimming pool looks about a quarter of the size as the one at my preferred hotel. At least they have a free cocktail hour in the evenings. If we each drink four glasses of wine, the room will only cost us $320.

After the cocktail hour, where we each only manage to swill one glass of wine before the owners send us on our way, we walk downtown. It's further than we expect, so we choose the first restaurant we find. As I dive into the warm pita, delicately fried calamari, and Greek salad, Stacy scans the room. She keeps saying, "It's your birthday! Let's live it up," but that may be hard to do in this town. Sure, there are a ton of men, but they're all with other men, or they wear suspenders with their plaid pants and walk with a slight stoop. Not that I feel up to partying anymore tonight anyway. We got up ungodly early to catch the plane down here, then sat in the sun all day. What I really feel like doing is curling up in bed and reading.

Stacy wants to go bar hopping, so we compromise on one bar, then back to the hotel. The only bar we can find is a Mexican restaurant with live music. We take a seat and I nurse a margarita while listening to a very poorly covered "Margaritaville." Even Stacy has to finally agree, it's time to go.

We open the door to our room and see a bottle of champagne on ice next to the bed, which is covered with rose petals. "Champagne!" Stacy cheers. "And a card for you. It's from the hotel owners. That's nice of them." She pours herself a hearty glass and is about to pour me one, but I shake my head. "Come on, it's your birthday!"

"I know. That means I should get to do what I want. I want to sleep."

The rest of the trip goes the same way: Stacy trying to convince me to party with her and me being dreadfully tired. One night we agree to see a movie together rather than going out. As soon as the previews for the new James Bond movie begin, I think I'm going to throw up. I have a strange vertigo feeling and the room is spinning. I have to close my eyes for the rest of the previews.

I think I'm pregnant, but then again, I think that every month. I'm not about to tell Stacy before I tell Jason, and I don't think I can sneak off to buy an EPT without her noticing. I'll wait until I get home. While I'm at it, I'd better lay off the wine as well.

Jason meets us at the airport and as soon as we drop Stacy off, I tell him my suspicions. He's excited, but keeps saying, "Let's not get our hopes up." We buy an EPT and I race to the bathroom to pee away. But as soon as I do, I throw the stick into the sink and run out of the bathroom.

"You look. I can't do it. I'm too nervous."

"It hasn't been two minutes yet," Jason explains. "Let's give it more time."

And then slowly, as if something might jump out at him, he opens the bathroom door a little wider. He carefully walks over to the stick and yells, "Two stripes! What's that mean?"

"We're having a baby!" I jump up and down and hug him. "I can't believe it! We're going to be parents. I knew it, I knew I felt funny. I knew it was real this time." I rub my belly.

"Wow," is all Jason says, but he has a grin on his face.

"I think I just felt the baby move."

"It's just a bunch of cells at this point," he informs me.

"Oh, I thought I felt something." I do a quick calculation and say, "Hey, it's a love child. We conceived on Valentine's Day."

We both grin at the memory of making love on our futon and pretending we were somewhere exotic. It was the first time I can remember enjoying being intimate, rather than trying to rush the act in order to make a baby. Maybe I should start wearing camisoles more often.

And to think, I was pleased enough about proving Sonya wrong when I horrified her with graphic details of our sexy night. Little did I know we made a baby as well!

"WE'RE GOING ON A TRIP, Sweet Pea. Your first vacation," I tell the growing fetus in my belly. Within a day of learning I'm pregnant, I start talking to and rubbing my belly whenever I'm alone. I've even indulged and bought a couple of baby outfits at the thrift store. But I haven't told anyone I'm pregnant. Sweet Pea is still our secret.

We're headed down to the Washington coast with several friends for the weekend. It sounds all well and good, except this particular group of friends takes drinking and smoking pot very seriously. And they expect the same from all in attendance. We don't want them to suspect I'm pregnant, so Jason and I spend the majority of the four hour drive concocting a plan.

"We'll buy some canned beer. That way you can carry around empty containers and no one will know the difference," Jason suggests.

"You expect me to drink people's backwash? That goes beyond the call of duty."

"No, no. We'll pour most of it out or I'll drink it and you can nurse half of a beer. Once they've had a few drinks, they'll stop noticing what you're doing, so you can stop pretending then."

"All right. And let's buy some gin and tonic too and I'll pretend I'm drinking those, but really leave out the gin. That way at least I'll get to drink something besides flat, cheap beer."

Once we're all there, I have a few sips of beer, realize it doesn't even taste good, so move on to tonic water. I plan on abstaining from alcohol for the first trimester and then see how I feel after that.

As the night progresses, the air becomes thicker with cigarette and pot smoke and the voices become louder.

"One more game of 'Screw your neighbor'?" Chris pleads.

"We've been playing that forever, let's play something different," Cami retorts.

In between coughs, Kevin agrees with Cami and gets up to enter the kitchen. "Anyone need anything?" he asks.

A chorus of "nos" follows, but I go with him anyway. I notice Kevin is drinking almost as slowly as I am and I ask him if he feels all right.

"Yeah, I have this cough that's hanging on forever. And my allergies are really kicking in. The owners of this place must have pets."

"Yeah, I smell dog. I think I remember that it's a 'pet friendly' house. Sorry about that, you must feel like crap."

"Yeah, I do. But the doctor gave me some codeine cough syrup, so I'll take some of that later tonight and sleep like a baby."

We both pour ourselves a glass of water and go back to the living room. Everyone continues playing card games and I say good night. A couple of hours later I wake up to the sound of groaning. It takes me a minute to remember where I am. The room is completely dark, due to no light pollution from the city. The groans are muffled and strange, but I assume it's Jason.

"What's wrong?" I ask his shadowy figure.

"My chest really hurts and it's hard to catch my breath."

"What do you mean?" I fumble around for a light.

"We were walking on the beach and all of a sudden, I couldn't breathe. I thought I was going to throw up."

"We need to go to the doctor. Maybe you're having a heart attack." I jump out of bed and walk towards the door.

"No, no. I'm sure it's nothing. Let me rest for a bit."

I watch Jason writhe around on the bed and clutch his chest. He's ghostly pale and his eyes are dilated. "This is crazy, I'm calling 911." I run down the stairs. Everyone is still up partying, but they don't even notice me. I find the phone, call 911, and start to explain Jason's symptoms. He staggers down the stairs as I talk. He barely makes it to the bathroom, vomits, and continues to clutch his chest. Every time I look at him, he grimaces and says, "I'm sorry."

The 911 operator fires away a million questions, most of which I don't know the answer to. Fortunately, Kevin has seen us and is now standing next to Jason in the bathroom.

"When did this start?" I ask.

"When we were running on the beach, he said his chest hurt. I guess that was about an hour ago," Kevin answers. He pats Jason's back when he throws up again.

I glance at the clock and tell the operator, "Around three a.m."

I search around for an address to give to the operator, but can't find anything. I don't even know what town we're in. There were very few signs as we drove here. All I saw was a large expanse of beach. Kevin finds the rental agreement hanging on the fridge and hands it to me. Meanwhile, I try to eke out any information from Jason.

The operator asks us if he has eaten anything strange. As I list all of the food and alcohol he consumed, Kevin asks, "Do you think it was the pot?" I cover the phone so the operator doesn't hear and shake my head. "Everyone else smoked as well and none of you are writhing around on the floor in pain."

"When did you say the ambulance was going to get here?" I'm crying now and my hands are shaking.

"They're working as fast as they can, ma'am, but it's all volunteers here. You're in a remote place. It may be up to a half an hour."

"Half an hour! He can't wait that long, he can't breathe!"

"Did he have anything else strange to eat?"

I look to Kevin, because Jason can no longer talk and is panting on the floor.

"Wait a minute," Kevin says. "He had a sip of my cough syrup. The codeine stuff."

"Why the fuck would... Oh, never mind." I relay this news to the operator.

"Well then," she says. "It's probably an allergic reaction to codeine. Best thing to do is keep him as comfortable as possible until the ambulance arrives. And if you need..."

I see flashing lights in the driveway. "They're here!" I scream and hang up.

Suddenly, five men and women storm into the house. I relay as much infomation as I can, while Kevin helps Jason on to the stretcher. Chris, Marty, and Cami seem completely confused by all of the commotion and are oblivious to what has happened. I see fear on their faces, and can't help wondering if it's due to being caught smoking pot. The paramedics take in the scene of smoke, dirty dishes, empty alcohol and beer bottles strewn everywhere, but don't say a word. I try my best to convey that not all of us are high and drunk so they won't think Jason's ailment is only from drinking too much.

They lift Jason up off the floor as gently as possible and lay him on the stretcher. He looks at my tear-streaked face and says, "I'm so sorry. I'm really, really sorry." He squeezes my hand.

They wheel him out of the house and I hear him groan as they bounce over the threshold and jolt him down the steps. I know they're trying to be careful, but their inexperience shows.

"Can I ride with you? Please," I beg the driver.

"Well, we're pretty full, but…" He sees the tears falling down my cheeks and says, "All right. Bill, sit in back with the others."

I hop into the front of the ambulance and ask him how long until we get to the hospital.

"Aberdeen is about a half an hour away if we make good time, which we should this time a night."

"Half an hour!" I scream.

"Yes, ma'am, that's the closest hospital. But your husband will be feeling better soon. Once they give him the adrenaline shot, his breathing should ease up."

From the back of the ambulance, I hear, "How do these things work again?"

"I think you jab it into this leg, really fast."

"Like this?" a woman asks. I hear a whimper from Jason as she punches him in the leg with a long tube.

"It's not working," she complains. "The plunger won't go down to administer the shot."

"You have to take the cap off," the man coaches. "Now try."

"Are you sure there isn't a closer hospital?" I ask the driver, wondering if half an hour with this novice crew will put Jason in more danger than being at home.

"Aberdeen is the closest. But don't worry, they've been alerted that we're coming. They'll be all ready for us."

I try to look in the back to see how Jason is doing, but I can't see him for all of the bodies in the way. And I can't talk to him because every time I try my voice is drowned out by the chatter of the other volunteers. I finally give up and start chanting to myself, "Please don't leave me. Please don't leave me."

I don't necessarily believe in God, but at times want to believe there is some sort of higher power. And right now, I want that higher power's help, so I ask it to please look over Jason and not let him leave me.

Thirty agonizing minutes later, the ambulance pulls up to the emergency room and three nurses run out to greet us. I'm reassured that we are finally in good hands until I hear a loud crashing sound. I turn around to see that although there are five paramedics and three nurses available, only one paramedic is actually wheeling Jason into the hospital. The other seven people are talking to one another and walking ahead of the stretcher. When the lone paramedic turns the corner, the end of Jason's stretcher, where his head is, crashes into the wall. Guiding Jason's head myself this time, we enter an exam room. A nurse pulls the curtain closed, takes a look at Jason, and says, "We'll be back in a bit. Another accident came in."

The hospital is eerily quiet and I'm suspicious of this other accident. It's almost five in the morning and no one is around. Does it really take all of the staff of the hospital to attend to one other victim? *Is* there another victim?

After twenty minutes of waiting, I am beyond agitated. Sure, the adrenaline shot, no matter how poorly administered, seems to be helping Jason's breathing. But he's still incredibly pale and his chest still feels as if an elephant is standing on it. I leave Jason with Chris and walk around the empty hospital.

I can't find anyone, so I follow the only sound I hear, the television in the waiting room. Cami, Marty, and Kevin are all sitting on the plastic orange chairs, looking haggard and red-eyed. The bright fluorescent lights don't make anyone look good, but this motley crew would even look bad in natural daylight. They've all taken turns waiting with Jason in his room, but I can tell their patience is wearing thin.

"No nurse yet?" Kevin asks.

"No, this is ridiculous. What kind of half-baked establishment is this? You guys should go home and get some sleep. There's no use in all of us suffering here." I point to the unyielding chairs and three-year-old *Good Housekeeping* magazines.

"No, no. We want to stay. We want to make sure he's all right."

I stomp up to the receptionist and ask her again if there is anyone available to look at Jason. "They'll be there as soon as they can," she says, without looking up from her forms.

When I return to Jason, I'm relieved to see two nurses bustling around him. One of them is placing an oxygen mask on him and the other is taking his blood pressure. After reassuring him, and me, that he will be fine, the nurse with the cuff says, "Oh dear. You need to turn the oxygen on when you put the mask on, otherwise he can't breathe."

I look at Chris and mutter, "Where are we?"

THEY FINALLY RELEASE US FROM the hospital with a few Benadryls to take if Jason finds it difficult to breathe again. It's mid-morning by the time we get home, but no one seems to be enticed by the brilliant sun shine. We pull the drapes shut and crawl into bed.

As Jason and I cuddle in bed, he looks at me and says, "I'm so sorry," again.

"It's all right. I mean, you're fine now, thank God, and it …."

"No, I mean about the baby. You're not supposed to be stressed when you're pregnant and I just put you through hell. Do you think the baby will be all right?"

"I don't know, but at least you are. I kept thinking about how I don't want to do this alone. About how much I love you and how I didn't know what I'd do if you didn't make it. How if someone had to go, I didn't want it to be you."

"I'm so sorry," he says again, brushing away his own tears. "You shouldn't have to think about any of those things."

"Just promise me you'll never take codeine again."

"Never again. I love you."

"Love you too," I mumble before falling into a deep sleep.

The rest of the weekend is a bit subdued after the drama from the first evening. We still stay up late playing games and talking, but without the heartiness of the first night. Sunday afternoon, Jason and I drive home, triumphant that no one realized our secret, but weary from the adventure. I return to work the next day and relay the story to Jennifer and a few other friends. Once we've caught up with one another, I enter my office, close the door, and have a little chat with Sweet Pea.

While checking my emails, I see that Karen has set a date for a group of "interested parties" to gather to discuss buying *Women of Seattle*. I jot the date down in my calendar and start listening to my voicemails. But I can't get comfortable. My lower back is throbbing and it feels like I have menstrual cramps. I write, "Out to lunch," on my door, lock it, and lie on the floor with my legs propped up on my chair. This relieves some of the pain from my back, but my stomach is still clenched in knots.

Maybe it's from all of the stress this weekend. Or maybe I need to eat something. All I had this morning was a piece of toast. Or maybe, no…. It can't be something wrong with Sweet Pea. I stuff that concern into the farthest recesses of my brain and try to relax on my office floor. When my bladder can't take it anymore, I sneak to the bathroom.

As soon as I pull my pants down, I see drops of bright red blood. Panicking, I run back to my office to call the midwives. I have the same HMO as Nina and chose to go with the midwives she used. I call the number they gave me and after looking over my paperwork, the midwife says, "I see you're about ten weeks along, is that correct?"

"Yes," I reply, while resuming my horizontal position on the floor. She asks me to describe the feeling in my abdomen (menstrual cramps mixed with food poisoning), the amount of blood (similar to a light period), and the lower back pain (agonizing). She sighs and a long silence follows. Then she says the words I am dreading hearing, "You're miscarrying."

"No! What can I do to stop it?"

"I'm afraid there's nothing you can do. A large percentage of women miscarry in their first trimester and there's no way to avoid it. Sometimes, it just wasn't meant to be. Or perhaps the baby wasn't viable. Or…"

I cut her off and ask her what I should do.

"All we can do is wait and see," she sighs.

I hang up the phone and burst into tears. I try not to believe her words and tell myself Sweet Pea will stay with me. She wants to be with me as much as I want her. Even so, the pain in my lower back is too great to ignore. I give up on trying to get any work done, write "Gone home sick" on my door, and drive home. Once there, I leave a message for Jason and call the midwives a few times. One of the midwives on call is very optimistic and I cling to her every word. The other midwife on call has given up on Sweet Pea. After talking with her, I have to crawl into bed and curl up into a fetal position. I convince myself that thinking about bad things only gives them more power and validity, so if I don't think about the miscarriage, maybe it will go away.

Jason comes home and finds me hiding under the covers "Is there anything I can do?" he asks, rubbing my back.

"No."

"What did the midwife say?"

"I've talked to a couple of them. One is really sweet and hopeful. She says I may just be spotting and that if I rest, I could stop bleeding. The other has given up on Sweet Pea and told me to come in for a D & C."

"What's that?"

"They scrape my uterus."

"Like an abortion?"

"Yeah." I pull a blanket over myself.

"Are you going to do that?" he asks.

"No, I hung up on her."

He asks a few more technical questions but I'm too tired to answer them. I know he is merely trying to understand the situation, but the fact is there aren't any solid answers. All we can do is wait and see. Which I find impossible, so I go back to sleep and hope that when I wake up, I'll realize it was all a nightmare.

A few hours later, I'm still bleeding, but not heavily. The "good" midwife is pleased to hear this and says if the cramps and backache subside, it probably means I'm spotting. I find comfort in this and am finally able to get out of bed. I gather two white candles and say a little prayer for Sweet Pea when I light them. I remember the advice my Catholic childhood friend gave me about always beginning prayers with gratitude rather than a plea. "Thank you for allowing Jason to survive in Aberdeen and thank you for blessing me with Sweet Pea. I know I've been asking for a lot lately, but please let Sweet Pea be all right."

I walk over to the window and look for a star. Ever since I was a little girl, I've been making wishes on the first star I see at night. "Star light star bright, the first star I see tonight. I wish I may, I wish I might have this wish I wish tonight." I close my eyes and will Sweet Pea to stay with me.

After another day of intermittent bleeding, the "good" midwife convinces me to get my blood drawn so she can check my hormone levels. "It will be good to know either way," she convinces me. I write down the directions to the after hours lab and wait in various cubicles to have my blood drawn. Once the procedure is over, I ask when I will know the results.

"Monday morning," the technician responds.

"But that's two days away!"

"Yup, we don't do labs over the weekend."

It's the worst two days of my life. When I feel all right and am not bleeding, I continue my talks with Sweet Pea. When my back throbs and I see blood in the toilet, I cry and crawl back into bed. And no matter what the situation, I light my candles and place my hand on my belly as a way to protect Sweet Pea. First thing Monday morning, I call the lab.

A cheery nurse says, "Oh yeah, here's your chart. Everything looks fine."

"Thank God!" I race upstairs to tell Jason and get myself ready for work.

I pretend I had the flu for a few days and no one seems to question my story. I work on the newsletter that it has taken me far too long to complete until I remember that I missed my first prenatal appointment with the midwives during all the drama. The receptionist asks me to hold for a moment when I call the office to reschedule. The "bad" midwife comes on the line and says, "Corbin, are you trying to schedule a D & C?"

"Why would I do that?"

"Didn't the lab call you?" she asks.

"Yeah, I called them. The nurse said everything is fine."

Long, long pause.

"I don't know why she would say that. I have your chart right in front of me. You're not pregnant anymore, you miscarried."

I stagger at her words and sit down on the floor. The room is spinning and I have to shake my head to clear it.

"No, I didn't. I hardly bled at all and the cramps went away after a few days. I'm still pregnant. I know I am, I feel it." Instinctively, my hand rests on my belly and I start to rub it in a circular motion. I'm sure the midwife is wrong and wish she would put the receptionist back on so I can make my damn appointment.

"No dear, you're not. Sometimes our bodies aren't aligned with our brains. Your brain may think you're still pregnant, but I can tell by looking at your hormone levels that you aren't. Now about that D & C. You really should come in and have it soon. Otherwise you may get an infection that could…"

Click.

I hang up the phone and lie on the floor again. Once the room stops spinning, I stagger into Jennifer's office. "I've been trying to have a baby forever and was pregnant, am pregnant, I don't know. I bled, but not that much, one nurse told me I'm fine but the other one says no, I lost the baby, but I don't think I did. I still feel Sweet Pea, I know she's still with me…."

Jennifer deciphers some of my babble and calls the midwives herself. Upon hearing the same news, she asks for more details of the story.

"If your doctor is the one who first validated your pregnancy, then she is who I should call. What's her name?"

I cry on Jennifer's floor while she tries to penetrate the impenetrable medical system. No one wants to answer her questions or tell her how or why I would have been told I'm still pregnant if I'm not. Everyone refers her to someone else. After the tenth phone call, I say, "Don't call anyone else. It's over."

I CALL JASON FROM JENNIFER'S OFFICE and then leave work for the day. I try to think of some excuse to write on my board, but Jennifer says, "Don't even worry about that. I'll take care of it. And don't come back for a few days, all right?" I nod and shuffle to my car.

Jason pulls up a few minutes after me, full of questions. I tell him I can't answer them, that in the end it doesn't really matter, and crawl into bed.

He follows me. "I'm sorry, you're right. It's just... I thought everything was fine. You weren't bleeding and the nurse said you were all right. Sorry, there I go again."

"It's hard not to." I snuggle deeper into the comforter.

"Do you think it was from stress? From the trip to the hospital and codeine?"

"I don't know. The midwife says not to get too wrapped up in 'what went wrong' scenarios. She says no one knows what causes miscarriages, they just happen. And they happen to twenty five percent of women."

He stares at his hands. "I can't help thinking it was my fault, that having you...."

"You don't know that, so don't kill yourself with guilt. I knew on that hell ride to the hospital who I was praying for, who I didn't want to leave me. If I had to choose again, I'd still choose you. Now get out of here, I'm going to sleep."

A few hours later, Jason shakes me gently. "Hey, are you awake?"

"No, go away." I bury my head in the pillow.

"Your dad's on the phone."

"Take a message."

"He wants to talk to you. He has some bad news. Your grandmother just died."

"What!" Now I'm wide awake. I sit up in the bed and Jason passes me the cordless phone.

"Dad? What happened?"

"She choked at lunch and they weren't able to revive her in time. She's had a series of strokes and they think perhaps that's what happened, but they don't really know. Not yet."

My grandmother hadn't been herself for years. Her dementia worsened until they started calling it Alzheimer's. Once she had to move out of her own home and into a facility, she deteriorated rapidly. She loved her home and had lived in it for sixty odd years. She repeatedly broke out of her nursing home and was found on the road "going home" in her night gown.

I knew she wasn't doing well, but I didn't think she was going to die soon. I had been thinking about her around her birthday, Valentine's Day. When I realized the baby had been conceived on her birthday, I liked the idea that my grandmother would have a kindred spirit. Someone who shared her special day. But now neither one of them will ever meet each other. Nor will I ever see them again.

I start to cry again and don't understand why my father is talking about Minnesota. "Huh?"

"Oh, you don't like Minneapolis. All right, you could take the Delta flight and go through Cincinnati getting you into Philadelphia around ten o'clock. That's pretty late, because it's an hour's drive to Grandma's, but..."

"What are you talking about, Dad?"

"The funeral. It's on Friday. You're coming, right?"

The last thing I feel like doing right now is getting on a plane and being around a bunch of people. It's a rare occasion that my father asks me to do something for him, so I feel as if I should be there to support him. But at the same time, I don't plan on getting out of bed this weekend much less flying three thousand miles across the country.

"I don't know, Dad, I'm not doing very well and it's awfully short notice." I wonder if I should tell him what's going on or make up an excuse for not attending. He doesn't even know I was pregnant because I was waiting to tell them in person when they came to visit in May. Finally, I just blurt out, "Dad, I had a miscarriage."

"Oh shit, I'm sorry." He offers more condolences and then puts my mother on.

"Don't say it," are the first words out of my mouth. I clearly remember the story about my mother miscarrying and her father, an Ob-Gyn, telling her, "That's all right, you're just priming the pump." My mother may have taken consolation in those words, but I don't. My body is not a pump and my baby wasn't water.

She tries to make me feel better by saying it's probably for the best, I'll have another baby, there's still time—none of which makes me feel better.

"I have to go," I tell her after a long silence. "Tell Dad I'm really sorry about Grandma and I'm really sorry I can't come to the funeral, but I...I... I just can't." I hang up the phone, crawl back into bed, and cry some more. I cry for my father, who lost his mother, I cry for my grandmother, who choked on her lunch and died, and I cry for my baby, who I never got to meet. I see my white candles, burnt down to a nub, and feel defeated. All that praying and hope didn't get me anywhere. Not only did I lose who I was praying for, I lost someone else as well.

AND THAT'S PRETTY MUCH WHERE I stay for the entire weekend. I tell Jason to make up an excuse if anyone calls for me and spend the majority of my time reading and sleeping. We take a walk and eat together, but even when we're together, we're both alone in our own thoughts.

I dread going back to work, but once I'm there, it proves to be a relief to have a distraction from my sorrow. I feign interest in some meetings, try to organize my files and office for whoever will come and replace me some day, and spend a lot of time staring off into space. I make it through the week and spend another weekend hiding in bed.

Although the midwife urged me not to, I can't help going down the "What went wrong?" path. I guiltily remember the margarita and wine I drank on my birthday and wonder if that's why Sweet Pea didn't make it. Or is it a karma thing? Was I a criminal in a past life? Is that why I'm being punished now? Or is it for bad deeds done in this life, like when I stole a friend's boyfriend? Am I a horrible person and that's why I can't have what I want so dearly?

My grief shifts to anger, beginning with rage against the nurse, all pregnant women I see, and the higher power that I called on in my time of need. And then the rage turns inward and I curse my body for failing to protect and care for Sweet Pea. How can I fail at something that is so natural?

Any progress I made by reclaiming the tight camisole on Valentine's Day is lost and I go back to loathing and being ashamed of my body. I won't look in the mirror, put clothes on as soon as I get out of the shower, and wear the same baggy clothes day after day. As for intimacy, Jason doesn't even try. He can feel my rigidity when he hugs me, so he knows anything more is out of the question. I'm locked in my own inner turmoil and no one is invited to join me.

The only thing that seems to offer some solace is weeding my garden. Spring tends to hit Seattle early, or at least it flirts with us for a while in February, when green shoots start to reveal themselves. By mid-March many of the crabapple and cherry blossoms are in bloom and pink and lavender crocuses, bright purplish blue scillas, and yellow daffodils are scattered everywhere. It's May, and seeing as I haven't spent much time in the yard, the weeds have taken over. While weeding and deadheading my tulips and hyacinths, I remind myself that everything is seasonal. Everything that is born eventually dies, but new things sprout up in their place. And when all of this beautiful Zen thinking doesn't work, I go back inside and take a nap.

I've been reading a lot as well. I like being completely immersed in the characters' lives and being able to forget about my own. I visit the library frequently and pour over the chick lit books. I would normally scoff at this genre, but right now, it's just the salve I need. I know immediately that the girl will get the boy—there will be a few obstacles, but they will triumph in the end.

I've tried spending time with people so I'm not alone, but it doesn't seem to help. Friends always say, "Don't worry, you'll have another baby" or "Maybe it's for the best." I don't want another baby, I want Sweet Pea. And how do they know I'll be able to get pregnant again? Maybe I won't. Maybe I'm incapable of carrying a baby to term. That's the problem, no one really knows anything.

After weeks of grieving and raging, I decide I'm ready to let Sweet Pea go. I can't live my life in bed. I'll never know what caused the miscarriage and I'm driving myself insane trying. I gather all of the remnants that remind me of Sweet Pea and place them on my bed. The cute baby outfits I bought and pregnancy book Nina gave me, I put in one pile to send to my pregnant friend Jill. I pause while folding a yellow snow suit and instead of adding it to the pile, I hold it to my face and cry. It's too heartbreaking letting it go, so I keep it. I don't have to give everything away.

I find the nub of one of the candles I lit for Sweet Pea and the cork I saved from the champagne Jason and I drank on Valentine's Day. I buy a hosta plant and Jason and I plant it in remembrance of Sweet Pea. I dig a hole in our garden and we place the candle and cork in it and the hosta on top. We hold hands in silence for several minutes and let the tears fall. At the same time, we break the silence and say, "Good-bye, Sweet Pea."

"YOU'RE GOING TO SPEND all weekend out there?" Jason asks.

"That's the plan. It's a retreat," I say as I stuff my sleeping bag back into its case. While wallowing in my depression, I had completely forgotten about the weekend Karen planned for all interested parties. When I saw it on my calendar I groaned, but now I think it may be a good idea to get out of the house.

"Doesn't sound like a retreat to me. Sleeping on the floor and working all day on the weekend. That sounds awful. And you should be celebrating not working."

"Celebrating not working?" I laugh.

"Yeah, it's your last day at Fruitloop U. Don't you want to do something fun?"

"The whole thing was sort of anticlimactic. I mean, I quit months ago, had to hear 'you're still here' for six weeks, and then I'll be teaching that class for the BA program over the summer. I'm not really done with Fruitloop U. It's the job that never ends."

"Maybe, but you should have fun tonight."

"You're not helping, I already committed to it, so I can't get out of it. Karen says it's a beautiful property with horses and big green pastures. Maybe it will be fun. Or at least relaxing."

"Have you looked at this schedule? It's intense. By the time you would normally wake up, you'll have already been through a small group brainstorming session, presentation by someone named B.J., and..." He stops reading and giggles at the name B.J.

"Only you and your adolescent friends think of blowjobs when you hear BJ. It's a real name, you know."

"If you say so," Jason smiles.

I can't say I'm actually looking forward to this weekend, but after talking to Karen, I'm hopeful that it will be interesting. She has a way of making everything sound exciting and fantastic. Hell, she got me to quit my job and come work for her for a third of the pay and no guarantee of a future. Convincing me to spend the weekend in the woods, for no pay, was easy in comparison.

I pack my car with a small duffle bag, pillow, and sleeping bag and give Jason a hug good-bye. He wishes me luck as I pull out of the driveway. I head towards the freeway and pop a Peter, Bjorn, and John CD in. I whistle along with "Young Folks" and sit back to enjoy the drive. I come to a screeching halt as soon as I enter the freeway. Bumper to bumper traffic. I thought by leaving at four I would avoid this, but looks like everyone had the same idea. Seattle traffic is notoriously bad, especially on Fridays.

I come to the 520 exit, the road that I need to cross over Lake Washington to get to the eastside, and quickly see that it's bumper to bumper as well. I crawl over the bridge and am relieved to see the further east I go, the more the traffic thins out. People get off at the Mercer Island exits, the Bellevue and Kirkland exits, but I keep on going. I think about Lydia and her son when I pass their exit. It's been months since I've seen them. Although I feel guilty about this, I know I won't see them anytime soon either. It's too hard to be around other babies, when I can't have my own.

I find my exit, and wind through a few suburbs. Not dense suburbs like the ones I already passed in Lydia's neighborhood, but rather fields and open spaces mixed in with developments. Eventually the tract homes and developments give way to green pastures with barns. The roads aren't clearly marked, but I find the dirt road I'm supposed to take. I follow it, pass a few horses staring at me with bored indifference, and arrive at a large white house.

I immediately start thinking of escape plans. *I'll stay for the evening, but not spend the night, claiming I can't sleep in strange places. Or I could leave now, before anyone sees me, and say I never found it.*

"Hey, Corbin. I see you found it all right," a cheery voice calls. It's Faith, Karen's twin sister.

Damn, no escaping now. "Hey, Faith. Yeah, the directions were great."

"Come on inside, almost everyone is here."

"Uh… OK. I'll meet you in there after I get all of my stuff." I'm still hoping for a last minute escape.

"I'll help you." She opens the door to the back seat and it squeaks and groans in agony. The seats of my fifteen-year-old Volvo are torn. Leaves, gravel, dirt, coffee cups, and pens and paper are strewn everywhere. "Looks like the inside of my car," she laughs. She grabs my bag and heads across the gravel driveway towards a door painted bright purple.

As soon as I enter the house, I hear women's laughter and smell an amazing mixture of aromas. Garlic, basil, and something sweet. I pass through the mudroom, full of twenty or thirty pairs of shoes in every size and color, and enter the kitchen. I see two bubbling lasagnas cooling on the counter, a woman slicing up loaves of garlic bread, and another woman tossing fresh greens in a huge salad bowl. Another woman peeks into the oven, announces that the pie crust is browning already, and asks where the tinfoil is.

Faith has disappeared with my stuff, but I don't seem to be able to leave the kitchen to go look for her. The woman tossing the salad smiles and says, "You look like you need a glass of wine."

"That would be great. I'm Corbin," I say, extending one hand to her and accepting a glass of wine with the other.

"I'm Susan, nice to meet you. Everyone is in the living room if you want to head on in."

When I don't move, she says, "Or you're welcome to hang out here for a bit."

I smile gratefully and ask if I can help.

"Maybe in a few minutes when we start serving. For now, why don't you just sit down and relax. I'm sure the traffic was grueling."

I sit down on a stool at the counter and watch the three women bustle around the kitchen. My shoulders relax and my body grows warm from the heat of the oven as well as the Syrah I'm drinking. As they start slicing into the cheesy, rich lasagna, I think, *Maybe this won't be so bad after all.*

ONCE EVERYONE HAS FINISHED their second or third helping of lasagna, bread, and salad, we get up and start cleaning. Half of the women head towards the kitchen and half head towards the living room. Food is put away, dishes are washed, and counters are wiped down in record time. The kitchen crew heads into the living room where the other women have moved the furniture to the perimeter of the room in order to clear space for our large group.

A table with coffee, tea, and pie is set up in a corner and everyone is instructed to sit down in a circle. Karen gives some background information on the paper, explains that we have all shown an interest in some fashion, and explains how the weekend will progress.

"But first, I think it's important that we all know something about one another. I have the advantage of knowing all of you, but most of you have never met before. Let's take some time to introduce ourselves, tell us how you see yourself contributing to the paper, a few lines about yourself, and anything else you think we should know."

I am thankful not to be sitting near Karen so I don't have to start. I never know how to boil myself and my life down to three or four sentences. One brave soul starts and after talking briefly about how she knows Karen, she describes how her head injury left her unable to walk, talk, or remember any of her loved ones. After years of therapy, she has all of her mobility back, but not all of her memory.

Story after heartfelt story is shared. Most of the women are in their forties, fifties or sixties and have led very interesting lives. I start to feel self conscious about only being thirty one and not having as much experience as the other women. My life seems so ordinary and plain compared to these women and my work experience feels trivial and unimpressive. Many of the women own their own businesses and one woman was the editor of a Chicago paper for years. I'm disheartened to hear that she is interested in being the editor of *Women of Seattle*. I was hoping for that position myself.

When it comes to my turn, I have no idea what I'm going to say. My editorial experience feels paltry compared to the woman from Chicago and my life story seems dull and uneventful. As the room grows quiet and I see twenty sets of eyes on me, I find myself sputtering. "My name is Corbin and..... Well, I wasn't even sure I was going to come tonight. I've been hiding in my bed for several weekends because....Well, because I just had a miscarriage."

I explain my story and when my eyes well up with tears, the woman next to me pats my leg and hands me tissues. Every time I look up, I see nodding heads, compassionate looks, and even a few tear filled eyes. This encourages me to continue my story. Once I'm finished, Karen says, "Let's take a break, stretch our legs, have some coffee, whatever you need. We'll reconvene in about fifteen minutes."

Tracy, the only other woman in her early thirties there, approaches me at the break. She puts her hand on my arm and says, "I'm so sorry for your loss. I know exactly how you feel."

"You do?"

"Yeah, I've had three miscarriages. The last one was about six months ago. I was five months along."

"Five months! How awful. I was still in my first trimester. Had you already had an ultrasound?"

"Yeah." She makes herself a cup of tea. "It was a girl."

I feel tears well up in my eyes again. "I'm so sorry, I can't imagine."

"No one can, that's the problem. There's nothing to say."

"I know."

"But my story isn't nearly as bad as Faith's."

"What's Faith's story?"

"You don't know? Oh, well I shouldn't be the one to tell you. You'll find out from her soon enough."

Tracy and I talk more about our miscarriages, the horrors of trying to become pregnant, and the awful feeling of never knowing if it will happen for us. Karen ushers us back into the living room and we all settle back into our seats or on the floor. The woman sitting next to me says she isn't ready to go next, so Faith offers to go. At first she amuses us with stories about her two young boys. She explains her varied career as a doula, accountant, and day care owner. She grows solemn as she explains why doulas and midwives are so important and how the right to choose a midwife over a doctor is being challenged in Washington State.

I assumed every woman had the choice, but Faith says that Washington is unique and that most states don't authorize midwives to practice in hospitals, or at all. Insurance companies rarely cover them and if women choose to use a midwife, they have to pay out of their own pockets. And if something goes wrong and they have to transfer to a hospital, the midwife can't accompany them. In fact, they have to deny the help of a midwife, otherwise the midwife could be fined.

"Midwives perform such an amazing service. Even after my stillbirth years ago, I can't imagine having birthed my ten pound boys anywhere else besides my living room floor. When Scott came out blue and not breathing, my midwife knew how to deal with it. The cord was wrapped around his neck, but my midwife reached up me and released it…"

I can't believe how matter of fact Faith is. I can't talk about my miscarriage without crying and here she had a baby die. I've never known anyone who had a stillbirth and can't imagine how devastating that would be. Yet she survived and went on to deliver two more babies. At home! Even after one of them was born blue! I could never do that.

MY SCHEDULE WORKING FOR *Women of Seattle* isn't that different from my schedule at Fruitloop U, except now I actually work instead of pretend to work. Most days are spent talking to advertisers, attending marketing events, or answering the paper's cell phone. I guess I could find this type of Girl Friday work demeaning, but I don't. Sure, I was hoping for the glamour and creativity of being the editor, but maybe I can still fulfill the need for creativity by writing articles. I have a couple of ideas jotted down, but can't seem to find the courage to actually complete an entire article. I tell myself that for now, attending events, even answering the phone, is gratifying enough and once I gain more confidence, I'll give writing a try.

I love working alone and being able to create a schedule that fits my needs and routine. It's so rewarding being in charge of my day, rather than feeling as if someone else is. I don't have to set an alarm and can always allow for time outdoors, visiting friends or taking a walk. Seattle's weather in June is fickle, so when it stops raining and is sunny, I garden or go for a hike. If I need to, I work later into the evening.

The schedule is ideal, the work is interesting, but the pay…. Well, I need supplemental work. I was babysitting Estelle for Nina a few days a week, but that gig ended when they thought I stole her.

I've never been good at keeping track of time and arrived at Nina's house an hour after I was supposed to. "Where have you been?" she screamed at me as I started to explain what happened. She told me she thought we were dead in a ditch or that I had taken off for Canada. It wasn't until she had Estelle in her arms and saw that she was fine that she relaxed.

After apologizing profusely, I started to get in my car to leave. That's when Tony showed up. He had been driving around the city looking for me and was not as understanding as Nina was. He yelled and screamed at me until Nina was able to calm him down. Although I really had only lost track of time, I could understand how they would think I had stolen their daughter. It's not as if the thought hasn't crossed my mind.

After that fiasco, I know it's time to find a new job. But every time I scan the want ads, I think, *How will I fit that in with my* Women of Seattle *schedule? How will I fit that in with a baby?* "I can't" is the answer I come up with, so I don't bother applying.

I try to explain to Jason how it's hard to fully invest myself in anything else because I keep thinking, *What if I'm pregnant?* He tells me I can't live my life that way. I say, "I know, but it's hard not to. I mean, we've been trying ever since I got my period again and I hope it happens soon."

"Being pregnant doesn't mean you can't work. Plus, any employer will understand when…."

"Quit being so rational! I hate it when you do that," I scream.

"All I'm saying is that maybe you don't need to worry about that now. Let's just take it a day at a time." He tries to stroke my arm, but I yank it away.

"I've been doing that for months and I'm sick of it! Everything is great except I'm still not pregnant."

"It happened once, I'm sure it will happen again."

"When?" I yell. He doesn't answer me. That's the problem, no one knows when or if I'll ever get pregnant again. I've done countless tarot readings and animal card spreads with this question in mind, but all they ever say is, "Patience is the key." I was so excited when I pulled the Otter card, which stands for woman medicine, convinced that finally I was going to get the reading I wanted. But although I tried my hardest to shape the reading to be a sign that I would be pregnant soon, I had to admit that all it was saying was what all the other cards and people have been saying as well: quit trying to force things and let life unfold naturally. But I can't do that. I used up all of my patience the last time I tried to conceive.

"I should be taking birth classes right now and buying cribs, not buying tampons," I tell Jason. "Why are there so many women out there freaking out when they see the two pink stripes, yet month after month, I wish for that to happen to me?"

"I don't know." He put his arm around me and this time I let him.

When I wake up in the morning, I have my period. I don't cry. Instead, I slam doors and hurl pillows across the room. I'm furious at my body for failing to carry and conceive a baby, and pissed at whoever it is that is in charge of these things, for not letting me have what I want so desperately.

Once I'm through yelling "Fuck!" and stomping around the house, I make an appointment with Faith's doctor. She referred me to a friend of hers who is an acupuncturist and "intuitive healer." Faith claims she's a marvel and has helped many women conceive. I've seen her several times and the main thing she does is talk to me and then prescribe nasty tasting herbs; but I'm willing to try anything that may help.

During my last visit, she asked about my work. When I explained that I was probably going to have to start teaching again, she became very interested. I'm not sure why, seeing as I don't enthuse very much about teaching. I babbled on about my writing classes and said that I was always surprised to find so many adolescent boys in my class, because I assumed that teenage girls were more interested in writing than teenage boys.

"It's significant that you're attracting thirteen-year-old boys right now; think about it," she said. Then she walked out of the room. Almost like a prophet or Obi-Wan Kenobi, telling me something profound and then disappearing into the clouds. I didn't see how thirteen-year-old boys related to my infertility, but I vowed to give it some more thought.

At her suggestion, I've been charting my temperature every morning on a graph. When my temperature spikes, I'm ovulating. Those are the days I ravage Jason. Then I lift my legs in the air to give the sperm the extra advantage of gravity.

Jason doesn't complain or tell me I'm crazy. He wants a baby as much as I do. Even when he's tired or has other plans, he performs. He also doesn't say anything when he finds me sticking my hand up my vagina and stretching cervical fluid between my fingers. When I ask him if it looks like egg-yolks, he gives the question serious consideration.

My library copy of *Taking Charge of Your Fertility* says the secret to knowing when you are ovulating can be revealed in your cervical fluid. The problem is, I always seem to have an abundance of cervical fluid (the book says this will only be true when ovulating) and it always appears to be clear and stretchy. I may have to give up on the vaginal exams and stick with the thermometer. Probing one orifice a day is probably enough.

SUMMER TURNS INTO FALL and still no baby. I continue tracking my temperature and ravaging Jason when my temperature spikes. I still really want a baby, but don't feel quite as desperate now that I'm free from Fruitloop U. Thank goodness I didn't wait to be pregnant before quitting. I try to fill the void I feel by visiting friends or starting various creative projects.

Now that I'm no longer commuting to work, getting dressed for work, and bitching and moaning about work, I have a lot more energy and time. I've been writing in my journal a ton and even completed a couple of stories about my childhood. I jot down what I remember and make up the rest. The baby urge must be causing me to think of my own childhood, because until now, I rarely thought about it. In fact, I can't even remember anything until I was about eight.

Writing is satisfying, but I'm craving something with more color. I buy myself some water colors and paper and experiment with blending various colors. I notice each one has a mood to it. Lots of red feels like anger whereas purples and blues feel contemplative. I find some acrylics and add words to each piece. I have no agenda while painting or writing. I just let what comes, come.

I find myself painting small hands reaching up to a yellow full moon. I mix green and blue and paint a watery background. I pick up a red acrylic and write "See me" on the horizon. I don't know why I choose those words, they just come to me. The painting completely draws me in and I can't stop staring at it. I tear it from my pad and place it across from my bed so I can look at it every evening and in the morning. It's trying to tell me something, but I'm not sure what.

I move on from watercolors to wanting to make a mosaic mirror. Jason builds me a wooden frame and I buy grout and several plates and tiles to smash. Breaking things is so exhilarating that after I smash the purchased plates and tiles, I gather all of our the chipped plates and the extra tiles from our remodel. I have a huge mound of broken glass and ceramic, but I want more. After breaking a few coffee cups, which are not chipped and too curved to be useful for mosaic anyway, I realize I'm getting carried away. I couldn't possibly use all of these pieces and soon we won't have any dishes left.

I love having time for myself and these creative endeavors, but my bank account is perilously low. It's time to find supplemental work. After calling a few of my teaching contacts, I learn that an after school writing program in Ravenna still needs teachers. The director is desperate, seeing as the program started when school did, two weeks ago. She says I can have the position if I can start tomorrow. I put my mosaic away and start drafting a syllabus.

The last time I worked with this program, I worked with fourth and fifth graders. I assumed I would be doing the same and am surprised to find a room full of seventh and eighth graders staring at me. I immediately throw out my Harry Potter and "being invisible" writing prompt and rack my brain to think of what thirteen-year-olds are interested in. I have no idea, but somehow manage to hold their attention for the next hour.

When it's over, I can't wait to go home. Not that the kids were horrible, they were actually very creative. It's just that I forgot how taxing teaching is.

Once I'm home, I immediately wash my face and hands. But this time, my ritual doesn't quite satisfy me. I need a bath. I want to clean my whole body.

I remember Wendy's healer's words about thirteen-year-old boys and can't help but notice they have reappeared in my life again. And yet, I feel so uncomfortable around them, so I'm sure I'm not consciously drawing them to my classes. If anything, I wish they weren't there.

As the room fills with steam, I place my loufa and several bath gels on the lip of the tub. I turn the stereo on in the guest room and hum along to The Mountain Goats. I've listened to "Hast Thou Considered the Tetrapod?" many times without feeling anything, but today I'm mesmerized by the description of a young boy hiding in his room. He's trying to disappear and go somewhere else in his mind. I have a vivid image of what that other place looks like and start identifying with the boy as if I know him intimately. Because I remember doing the same thing as a child.

My bath is forgotten as my memories take me back to my red wallpapered bedroom in Southern California. The large aluminum window, that I used to sneak out of frequently, is open and a gentle breeze flows through the room. The bookshelves are full of stuffed animals I no longer play with and books I no longer read. I'm a middle-schooler now, much too old for stuffed koalas and *Little House on the Prairie*. Yet I can't seem to get rid of these things. I'm lying perfectly still on my platform bed with my arms crossed over my heart, staring at the ceiling. My mom enters the room and asks if I'm sleeping.

"No, just spacing out."

"Oh, OK. Well, dinner's ready."

She leaves, but I stay where I am.

I remember doing this frequently. Lying as still as possible, as if I was trying to blend in with the bed. I thought nobody could see me and would be surprised when someone spoke to me.

Just as I start to dismiss the memory as one of dreamy adolescence, I think of all of the time I've recently spent in bed. Lately, when I crawl into bed, it's not to think. I'm actually trying to not think. I'm hiding from the world, hoping to disappear.

What was I trying to not think about then? I was just a kid, it's not as if I had "real problems." Yet, I can't stop playing the song and identifying with the singer. Over and over again I listen to it and don't understand why there are tears falling from my eyes.

WHEN THE FIRST SNOW FALLS in January and I'm still not pregnant, I fall into a deep depression. I've never been a huge fan of winter and not being able to conceive only increases my desire to spend every day in bed. The creative projects no longer hold my interest and the only thing preventing me from sleeping all day is my work with *Women of Seattle*.

Almost all of the interested parties from our original retreat are still involved with the paper. Only three of us are actually paid for our work, but the remaining fifteen women serve as advisors. Rather than a "Board," we call our group the Wisdom Council. We meet once a month to discuss the expansion of the paper, future design ideas, and marketing strategies. These monthly meetings, along with the more frequent production meetings, provide me with much needed camaraderie and support. The women never ask if I'm pregnant yet, nor do they offer suggestions on how to conceive. Instead, they hug me when I walk through the door and offer me a cup of coffee. And for the next couple of hours, I try not to think about what my life is lacking and instead think about what I do have: love, support, and a fulfilling job.

After discussing our successful fundraiser in December and congratulating ourselves on not only raising money, but significantly spreading the word about our paper, we move on to discuss the February issue. The issue focuses on less commercial and syrupy forms of love. We have several articles from single women who, rather than bemoaning their lack of a partner, explain all of the other "loves" in their lives, including animals, children, work, and spiritual practices. Another article explains several tantric exercises to spice up a woman's sex life. Again, with or without a partner. One of our columnists explores her sexuality and plainly admits that at times she actively seeks out one night stands. Instead of berating herself for this, she asks herself questions.

Is it all right to sleep with an undesirable man just because I feel horny? Why is it easier to be forthright after drinking a few martinis? How can I ask for what I need sexually without feeling like a slut?

Faye, our editor, is uncharacteristically quiet during this meeting. While the others whoop and laugh and throw out their ideas, she stares off. She and Karen exchange several glances and eventually Faye says she has an announcement. The room grows quiet and she tells us about her ailing mother. "I'll be moving back to Chicago to help her. This is my last issue."

Women stand up to console Faye and pat her on the shoulder, but I'm fixated on Karen's and Faith's faces. We can't run a paper without an editor. Are they nervous? What are they going to do? Once the commotion dies down and people settle back in their seats, Karen thanks Faye for all that she has done for the paper and says we will all miss her. "I have a few leads on other editors, but as you know, our funds are very limited."

My heart races as I hear Karen talk about the potential editors she'll be interviewing. *Now is my chance,* I tell myself. *You always wanted to be the editor and you'll work for a really cheap salary, quick, tell her you want to be considered for the job. No, no, I don't have enough experience. They want someone seasoned, someone with years of journalistic work under her belt. But they know you and you understand the vision of the paper. Just say it. You'll regret it if you don't.*

The encouraging side of me silences the self-deprecating side by getting aggressive. *This is your chance to prove you're not passive. If you don't say anything now, they'll hire someone else and you'll be left with regret for not trying. Tell them, tell them, tell them. Come on! Open your mouth and say something.*

I take a deep breath and say, "Karen, I'd like to be considered as the editor."

AFTER TALKING WITH SEVERAL potential editors, the Wisdom Council votes on hiring me as the new editor of *Women of Seattle*. I think I won them over by describing my view of editing as helping the writer shape the story, helping her see where things need to be clarified or expanded, and working with her to make the story the best it can be. A midwife of stories, rather than someone who would slash and burn another's hard work.

Thus, my dream comes true and I am the editor of *Women of Seattle*. And I love it. I love working with the writers and I love working with words. I ask questions about intention, maybe rearrange paragraphs for clarity, and then email or call the writer with my questions and suggestions. It fulfills me not only because it's creative, but also because it feels like a huge accomplishment to have spoken my desires. Instead of letting the opportunity pass because I was too timid, I took a risk. Instead of being hurt by the risk, I am immensely rewarded.

The stories themselves feel like company and I enjoy having them in my home. Although working alone is one of the things I love best about my job, I enjoy the companionship of the writers and their stories as well. After spending a few hours editing articles, I take a long walk and relish having my thoughts to myself again.

And within a few blocks of my house, those thoughts usually return to my lost baby. I rarely cry about the miscarriage these days. But I do grow impatient and frustrated, wanting to know when I'm going to have another baby. I try to tell myself to focus on the positive areas of my life, but that only works for an hour or so at a time.

My parents call and say they want to take all of us skiing. This is suspicious on a few levels. I just saw them at Christmas and sure, they're retired and spend more time in airplanes and on boats than they do in their home in Ohio, but they usually visit exotic places. And Seattle in February is not exotic.

I'm also suspicioius because no one in my family has skied in over five years. Jason has never skied, and my last memory of skiing involves waiting in endless lines while my feet and hands grew numb.

Reassured that this ski trip will involve a hot tub, great food, and possibly a lot more sitting than skiing, I agree to go. I even feel excited as Jason and I drive over Snoqualmie Pass. It's an unusually bright and sunny day, which makes the snow almost blinding. Having fallen recently, the snow is still pristine and white. It's dropping in huge chunks off of the evergreens and some of the drifts look nearly five feet tall. I roll down the window to take a deep breath of fresh, clean air. *Yeah,* I think to myself, *a change of scenery is just what I need.*

A few hours later, I listen to the people in the condo next to us scream, yell, break things, and then yell some more. Maybe this isn't going to be the relaxing getaway I imagined. We learn from the caretaker of the condos that a group of young Russians have occupied the condo next to ours. Without informing anyone or paying for the condo, they moved in. The caretaker has turned off their heat and their electricity, but they won't leave. He stops by every half an hour to update us on his new plan. We haven't skied or even touched the snow yet, but we've been entertained.

As we watch from our living room window, six police officers, the caretaker, and three repairmen escort the Russians out. Once they're gone, Stacy and I climb over our joint balcony to inspect the damage. From our side, it sounded as if every piece of furniture in the house was thrown repeatedly against the wall. Once inside, I see that's pretty close to reality. Wooden kitchen chairs are split in half, the heavy kitchen table is turned over, and bits and pieces of dishes are scattered all over the floor. Stacy opens the freezer and squeals with delight when she finds two fifths of vodka.

"You're not going to drink that, are you?" I ask.

She ignores my question and continues her foraging.

I walk down the hallway towards the bedroom to see what else they destroyed. There are dings and scuffs all along the hallway and, when I reach the bedroom, I see the sheets and blankets strewn about. I approach the bed and see what looks like blood on the mattress. I gasp and run back to the kitchen.

"This is creepy, I'm out of here," I tell Stacy. She doesn't seem fazed and continues to look around. I hop back to our balcony and head immediately to my room. My dad and Jason are watching the news and hardly notice me, so I'm able to crawl into bed without anyone asking any questions.

I feel sick to my stomach and can't wipe the sight of blood from my memory. I keep telling myself that it's not that big of a deal. I've seen blood before, but something about the bloody bed is very familiar and disconcerting.

I try to read, to sleep, anything to take my mind off of the blood smeared mattress. When I hear Jason walk down the hallway, I pretend to be sleeping.

I toss and turn most of the night, until a different image comes to mind. It's a twin bed this time, not a queen like in the Russian's condo, but the same streak of blood is there. I'm about twelve years old, standing next to a bed staring, just like I was tonight. But it's not a stranger's blood I'm looking at, it's mine. The same blood is in my underpants and on my pants and I don't know how it got there. I had my period a week earlier, so it can't be that. I walk around in a daze and finally find a bathroom where I can clean myself up. The blood doesn't come off easily, so I sneak out of the strange house and try to walk home.

I never analyzed the memory before tonight. I remember kissing an older boy in a dark room and then seeing blood in my pants later, but I never thought about where the blood came from or tried to remember more of the evening. Since then, every time I see blood, I clutch my stomach and feel anxious. At Lydia's and Nina's birth and tonight, I feared I'd throw up.

I start to remember more and more of that evening years ago. I went to the party with my girlfriend Jenny after drinking copious amounts of witch's brew. Witch's brew was a combination of any and all alcohol that could be stolen from our parents. Gin, scotch, brandy, vodka, whiskey, it all got dumped into a Folger's coffee can and stuffed into my backpack for later consumption. We almost always forgot to steal a beverage that could mask the taste. Once we were out of the house and safely concealed behind some bushes, we'd gulp the rancid combination down in large swallows.

Jenny was able to steal some pot from her older brother as well, so we got thoroughly drunk *and* stoned. We made our way to the party where I found myself being kissed and then pushed into a dark room by a boy that I thought was cute. He was a very popular eighth grader, whereas I was only in seventh grade. Although I was nervous about being alone with him, part of me was thrilled to be the object of his affections.

The memory had only included kissing and then finding blood in my pants, but more of the details are coming to me now. I remember Rick pushing me down onto the bed, lying on top of me, and pulling my pants down. I remember saying, "Don't," and pushing him, but he just laughed and kept going. I felt a sharp pain, yelped, and hoped that it would end soon. When it did, and he crawled off of me, I told myself he had only fingered me. I had no idea what a penis looked or felt like, so it was easy to convince myself that *that* was not what had entered me. As for the blood, I tried to explain that as an odd period.

I never told anyone about the evening. Not Jenny, not my mom, not anyone. I assumed it was my fault. I was drunk, I didn't fight hard enough, and part of me even wanted his attention. I never called it what it was—a rape—even to myself. Instead, I tried to forget about it.

Nearly twenty years later, I lie in the rented bed next to my husband, crying. The physical act itself doesn't bother me as much as the years and years of silence afterwards. Although I keep asking myself why I didn't tell anyone, I know why I didn't. I blamed myself. I thought I didn't fight Rick hard enough, so I "deserved" it. I was sure if I told someone they would blame me for being drunk and "loose" as well, which would only make me feel worse. So the only option I had was pretending it didn't happen.

But it did happen. And perhaps other things have happened as well that I've chosen to repress. Am I ready to remember more? Can I share these secrets with others? If I do, will my worst fear, that they will blame me, come true and will I feel more ashamed? Or will people actually help me? Am I willing to take that risk?

AS THE WEEKEND PROGRESSES, stuff continues to get broken apart and thrown around. Not by the Russians, they're gone, but in my head. More and more memories come to me as if pieces of a puzzle are falling in place. And the puzzle is me.

The memory of lying on my bed spacing out and trying to disappear and the uncomfortable feeling I have around the thirteen-year-old boys I teach makes sense now. I want to bathe after being around boys because I feel dirty.

But I'm not dirty, I was raped. And rather than admit this to anyone, I tried to make it go away by disappearing myself. I'd space off on my bed and hope it would swallow me up.

Shortly after I was raped, I became anorexic, another attempt at disappearing. I overly monitored every calorie I ate and exercised like a fiend until I weighed only ninety-three pounds. I'm five foot seven. This not only allowed me to feel like I was in charge of some aspect of my life, which felt out of control, but it also allowed me to feel safe from boys. I didn't know how to say no to them, so I kept them away by being too skinny. I knew I would be more attractive if I gained weight, but I was afraid to be attractive.

While anorexic, my period stopped flowing and doctors told me it was because I didn't have enough body fat. I ignored them. Eventually, I fell in love with someone and felt safe enough to gain the weight back. I was eighteen and ready to have sex for the "first" time. I went on the birth control pill, surveyed all of my friends about how to have sex and what it would feel like, and prepared myself mentally for the big night. Contrary to what all of my friends told me, I didn't bleed, nor did it hurt. I was suspicious of this, but, again, chose to ignore the evidence that it wasn't my first time being penetrated.

The second time I stopped menstruating was after a massage therapist molested me. There is a fine line between appropriate and inappropriate touch during a massage, but when I confronted the therapist, he avoided me and offered no explanation. That's when I knew something was amiss. Soon afterwards, my period stopped. Once again, my mind was telling my body, "It is not safe to be a woman, certainly not a sexual one."

The massage therapist, the botched biopsy when I had dysplasia, and the rape were all physically painful, but what had caused even more damage is that with every situation, I didn't stand up for myself in the way I should have. I never screamed or yelled or caused a scene; I just hoped for it to end quickly. And then I hated myself for being passive. Scolding myself for not being more assertive has become a bad habit of mine, yet being assertive feels harder than living with the self loathing.

I DON'T MENTION ANY OF THE MEMORIES on the trip and even when we return home, I give Jason the abbreviated version. It still feels too risky sharing all of it with someone for fear of being judged and blamed.

"I remember kissing a boy, but had blocked the rest of it out. But on the trip, I remembered more. I think I was raped." I fill him in on a few more details, but start to feel uncomfortable when he reaches forward to hug me and say he's sorry. I shift the topic to pregnancy as a way to avoid his shock and sympathy. I don't even know how I feel about being raped, so it's a mistake thinking I'll know how to handle other people's reactions.

"I'm blocking myself from getting pregnant. Even if I'm physically able, I'm mentally stopping myself. I'm all fucked up."

"No, you're not," Jason assures me. "I think I should get tested. I know you think it's you, but I've been reading that the majority of the time, it's the male's problem. I'm going to call my doctor and see what he thinks."

"That's crazy. It's not you, it's me. You got me pregnant, I just couldn't keep the baby."

We argue on and on in this vein for a while until I concede. I'm sure that it's me preventing us from having a baby, but know Jason won't rest until he's tested. He makes an appointment with his doctor and a couple of days later masturbates into a plastic cup. When he tries to deliver his goods to the nurse, she asks him what it is.

"My sperm," he whispers.

"Huh?"

"It's sperm," he says a bit louder.

"What?"

"I jacked off so you could check my sperm count!"

"Oh." She laughs, letting Jason know she heard him all along.

The results come back stating that 94 percent of his sperm are deformed. The doctor thinks it's due to a prostate infection and prescribes Jason antibiotics. Jason tries to have a positive outlook, saying now we'll be able to conceive, but I can tell he's only masking his guilt.

On one of our walks, I tell Stacy about the deformed sperm. "Oh, I always thought it was you," she says. "I thought your mind was interfering and once you stopped worrying about it so much, it would happen. You must be so relieved to hear it's him that's messed up, not you."

"I'm not relieved, I feel awful. I don't want Jason to beat himself up like I've been doing for months. It's no one's fault and I don't want him to blame himself."

"Maybe, but at least now you have an answer. He can take his drugs and then you can start trying again."

"I don't know. I'm pretty tired of the whole thing."

"You? Never! You're obsessed with having a baby."

"Yeah, but…" I'm not sure how to explain my feelings, so I keep my thoughts to myself. I know I don't want to have a baby in this state of mind. I need to take care of my own issues first. And if and when I'm ready to try again, I'm not going to do it in the same way. Jennifer's words haunt me once again. Obsessing about my cycle and procreating has been running away from something: me. I thought all my angst was about procreating, but maybe it was just about hiding from my past.

I concoct a plan for myself to find a therapist to help me deal with the rape, putting baby making on hold while I take some time to take care of myself. And when we resume thinking about having a baby, I'll do so in a completely different manner.

I call several friends and get referrals for therapists. Then I look for Jason to tell him what I've decided. I hear ACDC blasting from the basement and follow the noise. Whenever the vinyl comes out, I know he's depressed. The Clash replaces ACDC and he doesn't hear me approach him. I touch him on the shoulder and he jumps. When I explain what I've been thinking, he becomes angry.

"I can't believe you're giving up. What about what I want?"

"I'm not giving up, I just don't want to bring a baby into the world like this. I'm just suggesting we take a break for a while. It's gotten way out of hand."

"But I still want a baby."

"Good. Me, too. But for now, I don't want to focus on it. I need to get myself healthy first."

After more debating, he finally grumbles, "All right." He takes the Clash off the turntable and puts XTC on. I sit next to him on our lumpy beanbags and take a swill of his beer. Our arms are touching, but we're alone with our thoughts. "Dear God" is speaking the words we're thinking, so there's no need to speak: "…I can't believe in, I won't believe in you."

I STOP CHARTING MY TEMPERATURE, cancel my appointments with Faith's magic healer, and stop reading about fertility. But that doesn't mean I stop wanting to have a baby. After studying my menstrual cycle for over a year, I still have a good idea when I'm ovulating. And it's hard not to initiate sex during that time.

Jason's doctor claims it could take a couple of months for Jason's infection to clear and for his sperm to no longer be affected. That helps take some of the pressure off, seeing as he's firing blanks anyway. I try to use the time to start viewing my body in a more positive light, not as something that has failed. But I can't do it on my own, so I call the therapists my friends recommended.

After interviewing several, I decide on Vicky. She's in my neighborhood and I feel at ease with her immediately. I'm told she doesn't mess around and is tough and I view that as positive. I try to tell her my whole life story at our first session. She interrupts me and says, "Breathe. Take another breath. And another. Do you realize you haven't stopped to breathe once since you've been here?" When I say no, she says, "We're going to work on that. I see you can fill this whole room with words, but in doing so, you're not feeling anything. You're just talking. We want more feelings, less words. Breathing will help with that."

Throughout the session she stops my ramblings and says, "How does that make you feel?" When I answer with a thought, not a feeling, she points it out to me. "You've become disassociated from your body. It's a protective measure you've adopted, probably after being raped. It's understandable and quite common. What we're going to work on is bringing you back into your body. All right?"

"All right," I agree.

I trust Vicky and feel a huge relief by coming to see her. For the first time, I'm letting someone help me. I let all of my demons out and dump them on her office floor. *Here they are, make them go away.* But she doesn't make them go away, she makes me face them. And then she leads me to more demons, ones I didn't even know I had. When I try to avoid her or my feelings, she calls me on it. I learn to pay more attention to my stomach and less to my mind. My mind can tell me I'm fine, but if my stomach feels tense, I know I'm fooling myself. Rather than avoid that feeling, I stop and try to figure out what is triggering it.

When my birthday approaches in March, I start to feel sorry for myself and want to crawl back in bed. Last year, I was pregnant on my birthday. If I hadn't miscarried, I'd be carrying a baby around right now.

Vicky teaches me that when I feel depressed to go into it, rather than try to avoid it. "Don't try to distract yourself with projects, just let yourself feel your feelings. Let the emotions and memories come. You tend to try to stay busy, or go to sleep, as a way to avoid or control your feelings. But it doesn't work that way. You get sick or become depressed. You have to learn how to work with your feelings rather than fight them."

I let myself crawl into bed, but I don't hide from my feelings. I grab my journal and write and write. I write as much as I can remember of the rape and let myself mourn that my first sexual experience was a violent one. I cry for the little girl who felt so alone and ashamed, she kept the crime a secret, even from herself. I look at pictures of myself from that time to remember how young I was. As a way of blaming myself, I've always imagined myself older, savvier than I really was. I was only twelve, just a little girl, not someone who "asked for it."

I follow Vicky's suggestion of writing with my left hand as a way to let my intuition override my analytical brain. Writing with the left hand accesses the right, or intuitive, side of my brain. Plus, the handwriting looks like a child's so I view it as a way to access the little girl I've ignored all of these years. Remembering the little boy I identified with from the Mountain Goat song, I write the opening lyrics, "I am young and I am good." I write it over and over again, hoping if I write it enough, I'll start to believe it. And then maybe I can stop trying to disappear into my bed.

AS THE DAYS PASS, I START to feel better and decide to throw myself a birthday party. The morning of the party, I rearrange furniture, prep food, and marvel at the fact that for the first time in years it's not raining on my birthday. It's actually sunny and in the high sixties, a miracle for early March. Jason walks in and asks if he can help. Next thing I know, we're in bed.

We don't "get down to business" right away, but instead linger over one another's bodies. I feel nervous about having my body observed so closely. Although it feels good, I can't help but try to disappear. Emotionally, my mind drifts away. And physically, I want to pull the covers over myself so he can't see me. I remind myself that I'm safe, I'm with my husband, who adores me and would never hurt me. I'm not with Rick, nor am I a little girl. I don't have to do anything I don't want to do and I can stop this at anytime.

Once I relax and feel secure, I actually start enjoying the attention Jason is giving to my breasts. But once he travels further south, I tense.

"Are you all right?" he asks.

"Yeah, but don't touch me down there. Stay up here, all right?"

"Of course."

He doesn't seem insulted by my refusal of cunnilingus, so I try to not feel ashamed. Who cares if I have to call it "down there" or don't want my clitoris touched, at least I said as much. It's better than having him do so, as a way to please me, only to have me freak out or disappear into my mind to avoid the feelings. I tell myself to be proud that I stated my needs, rather than berate myself for refusing to be touched, but I feel a combination of both emotions.

Staying from the waist up feels safe and even proves to be titillating. I'm ready for him to enter me, and soon after he does, we enjoy perfectly timed orgasms. I can't believe how long I've gone without feeling desired, or feeling desire, and then satisfying that desire. While trying to conceive, I never cared if I was pleasured, I just wanted Jason to ejaculate so we could make a baby. And even before that, I know I shied away from intimacy. There were times that I disassociated from my body, even with my own husband.

As a birthday present to myself, I try to stay present through all of the sex and the snuggling afterwards. Jason obviously doesn't have the same goal in mind and quickly falls asleep. For a brief second, I consider placing my legs in the air. *No, I'm not doing that anymore,* I tell myself and join him in a nap. By the time I wake up, I see that the sun has gone down and our guests will be arriving in less than an hour.

I have a great time at the party and continue to celebrate my birthday for a couple of weeks after. I go out for dinner with friends, go to the Korean Spa by myself, and Jason and I spend a day downtown playing tourist. When my breasts become tender, I tell myself it's because I'm about to get my period. For days, I expect to see blood in the toilet every time I go to the bathroom, but it doesn't come. Three, four, five days pass and by now my breasts are in unbearable pain. It hurts when I laugh, run, even when I walk downstairs. Something is up.

I give it a couple of more days and then as nonchalantly as possible say to Jason, "Guess what?"

He stops mid-stride and stares at me with his mouth open. "No way, how did this happen?"

How does he know simply from "Guess what?" Couldn't that mean a lot of things? And what does he mean, "How did this happen?" How far back does he need me to explain? "Well," I stammer, "remember on my birthday, we made love and…"

"I know how it happened but we weren't even trying. I just finished my Cipro. My sperm are still…"

"I know, but I'm pretty sure I'm pregnant. I'm over a week late."

"Wow." He rubs his chin. "Did you get an EPT?"

"No, I wanted to do it with you."

We drive to the store and return with two tests, just to be sure. After peeing on the first one, I see two pink stripes almost immediately. Instead of jumping up and down, we both stare at the test. "Weird," is all we can say.

The shock wears off after a few minutes and I suggest ordering pizza as a way to celebrate. Jason smiles, but I can tell he's holding back. He's worried I'll miscarry again or that his antibiotic is going to make our baby have three heads.

"Nothing we can do now but wait and see. Let's get a large veggie with extra cheese, I'm starving."

I feel strangely calm as I pick up the phone to order the pizza. I know Jason's concerns are valid, and I wanted to take some time to work on myself. But I don't want to think about any of that now. I only want to bask in the joy of finally being pregnant.

I FLOAT THROUGH THE DAYS knowing I have a secret. I'm not ready to hear anyone else's opinion or concerns. I want to get used to the idea myself first. I want to take it one day at a time and not think about all of the "what ifs" and unknowns. And I don't want to get ahead of myself and buy any baby clothes or start planning the nursery. I'll have plenty of time for that. For now, I just want to be pregnant.

Eventually, I feel secure enough to make an appointment with a midwife. I don't even consider calling an Ob-Gyn. Ever since my dysplasia episode and the molestation from the massage therapist, I've vowed to only see only women practitioners. Not that there aren't women Ob-Gyns, but from my baby buzzard days I know that a midwife will spend at least fifty percent more time with me, will focus on my mental state of being as well as my physical state, and, since most of the practices are small, either she or her partner will be the one to attend the labor. There's no way I'm going to spend nine months building trust and a relationship with someone only to have a stranger show up at the birth.

I quickly learn that most Seattle midwives are only allowed to deliver babies in a birth center or home. I've changed HMO's since quitting, so I can't return to my previous midwives—not that I would want to anyway, seeing as they work in a group of six so I wouldn't know which one is actually going to be at the birth. It could be the mean one. I start to think that I'm not going to be able to have both a midwife and a hospital birth, so I call Afia for advice. She is a naturopath and midwife that writes for *Women of Seattle*.

"I have birthing privileges at Swedish and I'm covered on your insurance," she laughs.

"No way! When can I come see you?"

After setting up an appointment and explaining my miscarriage, I say, "Don't tell any of the other women at the paper, all right?"

"I won't say a word. It's your news and you'll share it when you're ready."

When Jason and I show up for our appointment, Afia walks us back to her office and props us up on a red velvet couch with zebra striped pillows. She hands us each a cup of tea and asks us about ourselves. Not sterile medical questions, but getting to know you questions. She explains her philosophy and her experience as a midwife and naturopath, tells us where she went to school, who she practiced under, and shares many heart-warming birth stories, both from in hospitals and people's homes. It feels more like we're in a friend's living room rather than a doctor's office. She never looks at her watch or makes us feel as if we are taking up too much of her time. She makes us laugh and puts us completely at ease.

When I ask her who will attend my birth if she's busy, she looks at me as if I'm crazy. "Wild horses couldn't drag me away from your birth. If I'm extremely ill, I have back-ups I can call, but that has never happened. I space my pregnant patients far enough apart so I can guarantee I'll be at every birth."

Jason and I grin at each other. I settle back into the couch, relieved to know a stranger won't be delivering my baby. Afia asks if there is anything else she should know about me. After a long pause, I say, "I was raped when I was young and am only recently remembering it. I don't know if that's relevant."

"Of course it is," she says. She moves next to me on the couch and takes my hand. "We'll address this as much as you want during your visits with me. I usually schedule at least an hour for each appointment, and if we need more time, we'll make it happen. It's going to be particularly significant as you get closer to giving birth. The memories may become stronger and I want to make sure you are prepared for that and don't shut down. Are you seeing a therapist?"

"Yeah, and that's our primary focus."

"Great. It's wonderful that you're facing the issue now."

I notice every time I tell someone I was raped, I feel completely numb. I don't cry or even feel sad while telling Afia, nor did I feel anything while telling Jason, Jennifer and Vicky. And I want the same reaction from the person I'm telling. When they show sorrow or move towards me to console me, I become rigid. I just want to state the facts and move on; I avoid sitting with the feelings.

Afia must sense this because she pats my leg and changes the subject. She asks if we have any more questions. When we shake our head, she says, "All right. Why don't you guys take some time to talk it over and if you have any further questions for me, you can always call. I'd be thrilled to work with both of you, but it's a big decision, so I suggest you talk to several midwives."

I look at Jason again and he nods, telling me what I already know. We're not going to look any further. This is the midwife for me.

III
First Trimester
Spring

First Trimester-Spring

"NOT AGAIN!" I SCREAM when I see blood in my underwear and in the toilet. I don't have the back pain that I had the first time, but the sight of blood is very disconcerting. I call Afia and describe it to her. "It's about as heavy as a light period and it's bright red."

"You're only in your second month, so it could be spotting. All we can do is wait and see if it continues. Try to rest as much as possible. Sometimes exertion will cause more bleeding. Do you want to come in and see me?"

"No," I sulk. "I think I'll take a nap."

I slowly walk upstairs to our bedroom and crawl into bed. Pulling our huge down comforter up around me, I try to escape my thoughts through sleep. But I can't sleep and anyway, I remind myself, I'm not supposed to hide from my feelings. I prop myself up with a lot of pillows and stare out the window. This time when thoughts and fears come, I don't push them away. I allow myself to sit with the fear and despair that I have around losing another baby. Once I stop trying to push these emotions away, they're easier to face.

Spending a week hiding in bed didn't prevent me from losing my last baby, so I refuse to do that again. I don't want to live my life in fear. I can't control what is going to happen by denying it. Sure, another miscarriage would be awful, but I'll survive. I've done it before.

I get up to edit a few articles, read my emails, and make lunch for myself. Every time I go to the bathroom, my heart races for fear of what I might see. The bleeding is lighter, which is comforting, but I'd rather it stopped all together. I walk outside to work in the garden and remember doing the same thing last year—although by last May, I had already lost the baby. I hope for a different outcome this time.

While weeding and deadheading, the blood increases. I scold myself for pushing it and curl up on the couch with a book. When Jason comes home, I tell him, "I'm bleeding again."

"No!" All of the color drains from his face. "What did Afia say?"

I relay our conversation, but he wants to talk to her as well. Once he hangs up, he announces he's going to drive to her office to buy some prenatal vitamins. Vitamins aren't going to stop me from miscarrying, but I know he feels as if he has to do something.

The week continues on in the same way. Every time the blood subsides, I breathe a sigh of relief, but then it returns. And when it does, I can't help but start to resent my body for failing.

"What's wrong with me? Why can't I carry a baby?" I ask Vicky.

She rarely answers these types of questions. Instead, she asks a question in return. "Why do you think it's your fault? You tend to blame yourself unnecessarily."

This quickly dovetails into the fact that not only have I blamed myself for the rape for all of these years, I also unnecessarily blame myself for other things. Vicky continues, "And by repressing the rape, you repressed the twelve-year-old girl inside of you. By keeping it a secret, you kept her isolated and trapped yourself with shame and unnecessary blame. You need to make peace with that little girl, to tell her it wasn't her fault and ask her forgiveness, so you can forgive yourself. She said no and that should have stopped the boy from going any further."

I nod my head in agreement. I know what she's saying is true, yet when I think about that little girl, all I feel is nausea, not love. Vicky sees right through me and says, "What's it going to take for you to forgive that little girl? For you to fully accept yourself?"

"I don't know."

"Fair enough," she nods.

I want to change the negative perceptions I have about myself, I just don't know how. I usually take a walk after my counseling sessions as a way to process all that was said. But walking seems to cause me to bleed, so I give it up. It's not easy, seeing as that's how I sort my problems out and how I clear the chatter from my head. It's my cheap therapy and I grow testy when I can't do it.

After three days of not bleeding but crawling the walls, I go for it. I take a long walk all the way to Golden Gardens. I walk along the beach, listen to the seals bark, and breathe in the salty air. Once I leave the beach and head back through my neighborhood, the fragrance changes from salt to lilacs. I pull several purple and white clusters of flowers to my nose and breathe deeply. I love spring, especially in my neighborhood, which is alive with color and fragrances. I cut several of my own lilac branches and some rhododendron flowers and mock oranges to bring inside.

I smile at my arrangements and feel very pleased with myself. Until I feel something wet between my legs. I brace myself for the worst as I pull my pants down. There's a little bit of blood, but most of the dampness is from a milky fluid. Although relieved not to be gushing blood, I wonder what the other goo is. Is it a yeast infection? Is something wrong with me? Why does it smell funny? And most of all, am I going to spend the rest of my life fixating on what's coming out of my vagina?

When I describe the fluid to Afia at my next appointment, she asks questions about its odor, color, and consistency.

"I don't know, it stinks and is more creamy than yellow."

"Stinks how?"

"Like, like…." All I can think of is vagina smell, but I'm not sure that's a medical term. Similar to many of the women in Eve Ensler's *Vagina Monologues*, I think my vagina stinks. Of all of the smells women used to describe their vaginas in the book, only two were positive. One woman said "roses" and another woman said "the earth." I love those answers, yet can't believe it about myself.

"Do you itch?" she asks. When I shake my head, she says, "Then it's not an infection, it's just increased vaginal fluid. You'll have that throughout your pregnancy. It's a good sign that you're progressing, but it doesn't stink, it's natural."

I'm embarrassed by my limited and derogatory opinion of my girlie parts. Why do I think it stinks when really it's just me? Vicky has pointed out to me how often I refer to my body in the negative. She claims my ritual of always washing my hands and face, or feeling as if I need a bath once I return home, is an attempt to cleanse myself from the rape. To me, the outside world is dirty. I'm only clean, or safe, once I'm in my home and bathed. And even then, I still feel dirty on the inside.

"ARE WE STILL GOING to your parents' this weekend?" Jason calls out the door. I hear him open a beer and throw the cap away. He comes outside, pulls a chair out of the shed, and joins me on the deck.

"I said we'd go out Saturday and spend the night. Is that cool?"

"Sure," he says. He reclines in his chair and closes his eyes against the late afternoon sun.

The last time I saw my mother was when I went out to lunch with her and told her about the rape. She, like Jason, asked if there was anything she could do for me.

"I don't know," I said. "But I think telling you is helping."

Even though I felt numb while telling her, I still think it was helpful to do so. It feels as if every time I tell someone, I dispel some of the power it's been holding over me. The secrecy has been a main cause of the damage, so by eliminating that, I hope to move towards healing myself.

I don't tell anyone else in my family, but assume my mom told my father about it, that being the way things usually work between us. We haven't discussed it further and as far as they know I'm taking a break from baby-making and working on myself.

This spring they started to look for a house near Seattle and recently bought one on Bainbridge Island, which is a thirty minute ferry ride from Seattle. I've lived thousands of miles and even continents away from my parents, and

I'm not used to the idea of living so close to them. Even harder to imagine is them being grandparents. They have friends all over the world and are used to jetsetting here and there. I don't think of them as being retired and settled, nor can I imagine them sitting around baking cookies or knitting baby blankets.

As soon as we arrive at their house, Jason and I try to tell them our big news. It proves to be more difficult than I imagined. I can't get either of them to sit down, much less stand still for five minutes. They bounce from room to room, showing us all of the amazing architectural features of their new house, hanging paintings, and rearranging furniture all the while. Exhausted, Jason and I eventually plop down on their leather sofa, while they continue to flit about.

"How are we going to tell them when they won't sit still for more than a minute?" Jason whispers.

"I know, they're crazy. I think they forgot about feeding us too. I was dropping major hints to my mom, like 'When's dinner?' and she just laughed."

"I'm gonna go for it." Before I can ask him what he means, Jason calls out, "Hey guys, come in here for a minute. We have some big news."

I hear my dad walk into the den to freshen his drink and my mom hangs another picture, but eventually they join us in the living room. Before they even sit down, Jason blurts out, "Corbin's pregnant."

"Hot damn!" my mom screams as she races over to hug me.

"That's great news," my dad says with a tear in his eye.

I don't know what I expected from them, but it wasn't this. I've never heard my mom sound so excited and I've rarely seen my dad cry. I get up to hug both of them and bask in all of their attention. I tell them how far along I am and about Afia. Just as I sit back and prop my feet up on the coffee table, ready to be admired, congratulated, and hopefully fed, my mom says, "It's great news, really it is. Now come help me scrub out the kitchen pantry."

The weekend continues in the same vein. Some celebrating, some cleaning, and lots and lots of bustling from my parents.

I keep all of it in mind when we meet with Jason's dad and stepmom the following weekend. Now that I'm past my first trimester and not as concerned about a miscarriage, we're telling everyone.

Over chopped salads at a local Italian restaurant, Jason blurts out the news again. Eileen hugs me and grins like a lunatic while his dad says, "That's great. That is just so great." When his dad's eyes well up with tears, I look at Jason with alarm. *Oh no, another crying dad.* I don't know how to deal with this. The tears only last a moment and then his dad pontificates about String Theory, his favorite subject.

Stacy and I take a walk together later that day. We're almost back to my house and I haven't told her yet, so I interrupt her work story with, "I'm pregnant."

"What? No way! When did that happen?"

"I'm almost three months along." I open my kitchen door and enter the house. I babble about the spotting and my fear as I open the refrigerator. I take a bottle of wine out and get ready to pour Stacy a glass. We usually hang out after our walks and talk and drink wine, but Stacy doesn't accept my wine glass. She just stands in my kitchen with her mouth hanging open. Then she says she has to leave. Which leaves me standing with my mouth hanging open.

I'm not sure how much more of this I can take. Everybody is acting so weird. It's not as if my pregnancy should surprise anyone. I've talked about little else for the past year and a half. Crying dads and exclaiming mothers I can understand. Sure, it's uncharacteristic, but it sort of makes sense. But a silent and shocked Stacy? I don't get it. Was she starting to think I was incapable of becoming pregnant? Is it strange for her to think of her younger sister doing something before her? Or is she just shocked that I was able to keep it a secret for so long?

PEOPLE CONTINUALLY ASK ME if I feel nauseous or have morning sickness and I proudly say, "No. I feel great. In fact, do you have any food on you?" I've already gained fifteen pounds and I'm only three months along. If I do the math, I could be concerned about this, but thankfully my hormones not only make math impossible, but also make me too blissed out to worry. Afia says pregnancy hormones are similar to being drunk, but without any of the negatives. She's right. I bump into things and am spacey, but always have a huge grin on my face. So far, I'm a friendly drunk.

Jason packs the car for our weekend in Portland while I accidentally knock things over and talk to myself. Once we arrive at Jenny and David's house, we try our hardest not to bore them with our baby stories, but I'm pretty sure we fail. Talking about the baby's heartbeat and what we thought was the amazing ultrasound earn us a few polite nods. I should have stopped there, but instead go on to describe the image of our little baby squirming around, flipping this way and that. "S/he has legs, arms, a huge head, and we even saw the heart beating. It was just like a commercial, Jason and I crying and holding hands while the technician beamed at us. I have a picture, want to see?"

They smile politely, but I see Jason shaking his head. I sit back down and say, "Maybe I'll show you later." It's so hard to act like a normal person.

Once we return from Portland, I take the ultrasound picture of our baby out and stare at it as much as I want. I look at the picture and talk to my belly every day. And then I stare at my boobs. Another beautiful reminder that I am indeed with baby. They're huge! I've always pined for larger breasts and can't believe Jason is unimpressed.

"Look at 'em, they're falling out of my bra! I've always wanted boobs like these."

"I know, you're crazy for boobs." Jason shakes his head and laughs, but somehow resists staring at them. I don't get it. I'm offering him a free show and he just walks away. Where's the enthusiasm?

Although I adore my new bosom and am happy to show them to Jason any time, I notice my stomach clenches when other men notice them. While walking past the deli, several men stop their conversation and leer at me. I feel my shoulders curl and I cross my arms across my chest. A second ago, I felt quite confident and pleased with myself and my cleavage, but one look from the men changes that to shame. And then anger. *Stupid men,* I mutter to myself. *Can't they see I'm pregnant?*

When I return home, I try on all of my tank tops to see if I have one that will cover my breasts more. I stop myself after the sixth shirt fails to act as a burqa. *What am I doing? I've wished for breasts like these my whole life. Screw those guys. I'm not going to hide because of them. It's my body and I can show it off if I want.*

My words sound convincing now that I'm home alone in my house, but I doubt I'll be able to believe them the next time I see a man leer at me. I look over at the watercolor I painted with the moon, hands, and the words "See Me." It's true, I want people to see me and validate me, yet am scared when it actually happens. I've spent years trying not be noticed, because that's what felt safe. And I still don't know how to feel comfortable being looked at, admired, or touched, yet part of me wants that desperately.

I take a little piece of paper out of my night table and write, "I am safe," on it. I stick it in my bathroom mirror where it joins "I am good." I hope by staring at these words every day, they'll be embedded in my psyche. And then, I can stop hiding and being afraid.

IV
Second Trimester
Summer

Second Trimester-Summer

JUST HOW MUCH CAN ONE barely employed pregnant woman sleep? After nine (or ten) hours of sleep at night, I'm still ready for a nap by one. And I can't even inject caffeine into my veins like every other Seattleite. After half a cup of coffee, I'm doubled over with cramps. The diarrhea that follows makes me swear off caffeine for the remainder of the pregnancy. I miss the drunk hormones, they were way more fun than the sleepy ones.

Similar to everyone else in Seattle, I'm used to packing as many music festivals, trips to the coast, outings with friends, and late nights as possible in our very short summer. The problem is that I have the energy of a slug. After one music festival, I sleep for two days. At first I resented my inability to remain vertical for more than four hours in a row, but then I balanced my checkbook. It's a lot lower than I hoped, so I may as well enjoy being horizontal. At least I won't spend money that way.

I was offered a couple of teaching contracts in the spring, but only accepted two. I think I slept through the other interviews. And now that it's June, the summer schedules are not only reduced, but set as well. I won't be able to teach until fall. Not that I mind not working, I just want the money. I can survive on my paltry salary from *Women of Seattle* as long as I'm careful.

I rationalize my slovenliness and alleviate my guilt for not looking for more work by re-reading my horoscope from *The Stranger*. It states, "You have a cosmic mandate to slip away from the vision-narrowing routine and climb to the mountaintop—or at least to a mountaintop perspective. There I predict you will receive the exhilarating benefits of viewing the big picture from on high. You will prune away all but one goal, pledge to devote yourself to it utterly, and formulate a step-by-step strategy to achieve total victory by December."

I tape this to the wall in my office to remind myself that I'm busy. Busy making a baby that's due in November. Between the therapy sessions, appointments with Afia, prenatal yoga class, daily walks, and sleeping ten hours a day, it's all I can do to work for *Women of Seattle*. I resign myself to a summer of cheap relaxation and tell myself I have the rest of my life to work more.

When I tell Stacy about my summer plan, she becomes excited about the working less part, but balks at the cheap or free activities I suggest.

"Picnics and painting your toenails are not fun activities. Let's do something exciting. Let's go out."

"I can't drink and I don't want to spend any money."

Click.

I guess I won't be seeing much of Stacy this summer. Ever since I told her about my pregnancy, I've felt some distance growing between us. When I talk about my pregnancy, which is frequently, she doesn't understand or she makes fun of me. You'd think I'd be used to her calling me obsessed—I lived with "baby buzzard" after all—but now it bothers me. It feels as if she's not only insulting me, but negating my baby as well. My maternal instincts must be kicking in already because I'm not about to let anyone insult my baby.

After a few weeks of not hearing from her, Stacy calls me. "I found a great place to camp, right on Lake Chelan. I booked it for next weekend."

"Cool, that will be fun."

"I'm coming over so we can plan the menus."

We buy out half the grocery store (so much for cheap), pack Stacy's Saab full of pillows, lawn chairs, air mattresses, sleeping bags, a cooler full of food, another cooler of beer, and an inflatable boat to loll around in. It takes both of us to close the trunk, but I feel confident that we have everything.

As we drive over the mountains, I tell her about my recent photo shoot with my friend Lori.

"God, you're so obsessed with your pregnancy. Why do you need to document every moment of it?"

I usually laugh at myself when she calls me obsessed, but this time I feel defensive. "Of course I'm obsessed! It took me years to finally get here, why wouldn't I want to cherish it? It's a life changing event. What do you think I'm going to do, ignore it?"

"The baby's not even here yet. Why do you have to do all of this stuff now?"

"Because I'm doing what I can to ensure that I've taken care of my issues and made the kind of life I want, so I can focus on the baby when it arrives. I don't want to transfer any of my unresolved issues onto my baby. And I want to make sure I feel fulfilled before the baby comes, so I don't expect it to fill any gaps."

"Can't you just take some vitamins and have an ultrasound like a normal person?"

"Sure, but that's not what I mean." I pause, not knowing how to explain myself to Stacy. I haven't told her about being raped, nor does it seem as if she understands why I want to get myself into the best possible shape—mentally, physically, and emotionally—before I have a baby. "Sure, taking vitamins helps, but I want to do more than that. Like the photoshoot with Lori. It was empowering to allow myself to really be seen like that. I was completely naked, but didn't feel self-conscious or ashamed ..."

"Oh God, did you and Lori strip and howl at the moon again?" Stacy loves claiming that the majority of my ten-year friendship with Lori has been spent getting naked and performing strange rituals. It's true, Lori is very spiritual and we have spent many hours reading tarot cards, holding dark moon rituals where we light candles and burn pieces of paper with things that no longer serve us written on them, but we have never, ever gotten naked and howled at the moon.

I don't have the energy to try to explain myself any further, so I change the topic. We enjoy ourselves for the remainder of the trip, but I continue to feel as if Stacy would rather I wasn't pregnant. Or at least is trying to ignore my pregnancy. She chides me for not drinking—"It's only Coors Light, come on, it's practically water"—and walks away when any of the other campers ask about my pregnancy. Unfortunately for her, I never decline an offer to talk about my pregnancy.

We are adopted by a group of adolescents and one of the boys seems to be particularly inquisitive. While the other kids set off fire crackers, blow Stacy's air mattress up for her, or push each other into the lake, Sean asks me about my life. He's fascinated to learn that although Stacy is older, she is not married, nor ready to have kids. He asks about our childhood and our relationship now, and then we move on to the pregnancy. I tell him all about my miscarriage, Jason's deformed sperm, and more than he would ever care to know about cervical fluid. While I'm in heaven talking about bodily fluids, Stacy calls out, "Quit boring Sean to death and come here. They're gonna teach us some hip hop moves."

I watch my sister boogey around in the dirt and can't help smiling. She doesn't want to go deep or discuss bodily fluids, she just wants to have fun. She may not understand my choices or even agree with them, but I know she cares about me. And even though I wish she would show that care in other ways sometimes, I still love her. She's my big sister.

I forget about our differences for the time being and get up to dance with her.

DURING THE REMAINDER of the camping trip, I give the cervical fluid discussions a rest and enjoy Stacy's company. When it feels as if she's being dismissive towards me, I wonder if it could actually be that she's trying to protect me. She has looked out for me my whole life.

Maybe she isn't being mean, she's just afraid. Afraid for me, or afraid to think about the issues I'm bringing up.

We swim in the lake, play cribbage, take long walks together, and, of course, are constantly entertained by the adolescents. Around eleven each night, we have to kick them out of our campsite so we can go to sleep. They seem to subsist on sugar and don't require sleep. When it's time for us to leave, I actually feel tears well up in my eyes as I hug all of them good-bye.

I return home well rested, well fed, and ready to get back to work. I've been working hard on editing the July issue and am looking forward to sharing the details at our Wisdom Council meeting. Once everyone has arrived at Faith's house and we have time to greet one another, we gather in the living room. I sit on Faith's couch, propped up by various pillows, ready to discuss the July line up with everyone. But before I have a chance, Karen starts to discuss some changes she and Faith are making to the paper.

"Faith and I have come up with a brilliant idea for summer. Funds are low, as you all know, so we're going to combine the July and August issue. If we have to, we'll even run it through September. That way we won't have to pay to print three issues, we'll just run a special extended summer issue."

I look around the room to see if I'm the only one that is nervous about this idea. A few women are concentrating deeply on what Karen is saying, but most of them are caught up in her enthusiasm. They're nodding their heads in agreement and smiling.

"That's really exciting," I interrupt, "but aren't you worried about how advertisers and writers will view this decision? They may be upset because they have timely events or news to share over the summer. Or they may view us as unreliable. We're not giving them very much notice. I already have all of the articles edited and ready to go and told the writers the paper will be out by the first."

Karen and Faith nod at what I'm saying, but I can tell they have already made up their minds. And then it hits me. Why am I so worried about the advertisers and writers? What about me? No August and possibly no September issue means no articles to edit, which means no paycheck. *Shit!*

My mind races with every possible contact I have for freelance work. Teaching is out for summer, but I could beg and plead for some work in the fall. Just how many directors did I blow off? Can I blame my pregnancy? Maybe I need to start scanning the want ads again. Oh, who am I kidding? Even if I could stomach a nine to five job again, which I know I can't unless I give myself a lobotomy, no one is going to hire an extremely large, forgetful, and moody pregnant woman. I'm so screwed.

Once the meeting is over and women start to hug good-bye and leave, I approach Karen and Faith. My palms are sweating with nervous anticipation. I'm horrible at asking for things, especially money, but this is my livelihood and I want to make sure that's considered.

"Um, you guys?" I start. Once I have their attention, I ask the dreaded question. "Will I still be paid over the summer? I cleared my teaching schedule and was hoping to make it on my salary from the paper."

They look at one another nervously, so I quickly add, "I mean, obviously I won't be editing as much, but I'm happy to increase my hours doing other things. I can go to more marketing events, or help follow up with advertisers, or whatever needs to be done."

I can tell I'm babbling and Faith relieves me of my discomfort by touching my shoulder. She smiles at me and says, "Don't worry. We'll work something out."

I breathe a huge sigh of relief. It's nothing set or clear, but that's the way it's always been with this paper. And so far, it has worked out.

PREGNANCY PROVIDES THE GET OUT of jail free card I've been yearning for my whole life. When I accidentally say the rude thought

I was thinking out loud, people just laugh. When I call past employers and say, "Sorry I never sent you my course description, it slipped my mind because I'm pregnant," they say, "No problem, just email it to me now. How many classes do you want to teach in the fall?" When I say I'm tired, Jason makes me dinner and offers to rub my back. I should have taken advantage of this months ago.

I'm reassured that I'll have enough work in the fall and now have to figure out how to make it for the summer. Karen and Faith are able to pay me a little bit, but it won't be enough to cover my share of the bills. Jason offered to work more, but then who would cook dinner? Plus, we decided years ago to never let money come between us. It's a surefire way to end up divorced. We have different spending philosophies and neither one of us is the breadwinner. We contribute equally to the household account and whatever is left over from our paychecks, we're free to spend as we please. It's worked so far and I really don't want to mess up a good thing. Thank goodness I have a healthy savings account. Looks as if I'll be tapping into it this summer.

With my money/work situation sort of resolved, I focus on my real work—making a baby. I've been winging it so far and it seems to be working, but maybe it's time for me to educate myself. Maybe I could devote one of the ten hours I spend in bed reading about pregnancy.

After an hour spent sitting on the dirty library floor pouring through pregnancy books, I decide I may have to buy a book. All of the books at the library seem antiquated, worrisome, or syrupy sweet. I don't relate to any of the women, nor do I share any of their concerns. Entire chapters are devoted to "What if my water breaks while I'm in public?" Lucky for me, I rarely leave my house. And after watching Nina and Lydia bleed, urinate, and defecate all over the place, I know that others thinking I peed my pants is the least of my worries. Besides, I already pee my pants and am quite used to doing so in public. Every time I walk and sneeze or walk and laugh, my underwear and pants end up drenched in urine. Afia says I have to practice my kegels, but here's another little secret: I hate kegels.

Everyone claims they are so easy and so important, yet I don't know how to do them. I try and try, but am clearly kegel inept.

I walk over to my local bookstore, hoping I won't sneeze along the way, and plop down in the pregnancy section. Again, I can't relate to any of the books. Most of them want to devote a third of the book to pregnancy and the rest is all about the birth. The birth is four or five months away, which feels like a lifetime. I want to know what's going on inside of me now, but most of the books seem to gloss over the pregnancy with a tone that says, "Don't worry about that, little lady." As if I don't have a say in it, so why bother trying to understand it?

None of the books talk about sexual issues and very few even mention midwives. They assume that a doctor will be involved as well as a hospital. And the more I read about hospitals, the more unsure I feel. Episiotomies, Pitocin, stripping membranes, inducing labor, and epidurals are such common phrases in the books, yet after five meetings with Afia, we've never talked about these things. She describes birth as a natural event, something that the woman intuitively knows how to do. These books all describe birth as an act to be managed and monitored. I don't like to be managed, that's why I work from home. And I don't know how I feel about being monitored either. Sure, I want to know the baby is all right, but I assume s/he is, otherwise my body would let me know. I would bleed again or stop feeling him/her move around. I've started trusting my body more and marvel at how it seems to be able to nurture and grow this baby without me telling it what to do. I feel the baby's kicks and beam. "I'm growing a baby!"

As for control, I'm learning through therapy that my need to control things is related to the fear that if I don't, I'll be hurt. Just like I was raped. But I can't control the pregnancy, even if I wanted to. I know women who have ultrasounds every month, just to be sure everything is all right. Sure, the ultrasound was thrilling and alleviated a lot of fear I had about miscarrying, but they aren't foolproof. Many disorders and maladies aren't detected by ultrasounds and, as in all things, there are no guarantees. I feel the tests give a false sense of reassurance to expecting mothers. I can't control what happens to my baby, but I can learn to trust my body and begin to view it as an advocate rather than a failure. I would rather rely on myself for a sense of well-being than a machine.

We considered having a second ultrasound to determine the sex, but once we discussed this option with Afia, we decided against it. I haven't known the sex thus far, what's another four months? Does it really matter? I have mixed feelings about both sexes. Part of me wants a girl, because that's what I'm used to. I rarely feel comfortable around men, prefer the company of women, and fear that my rape may cause me to resent or be angry at my son when he becomes an adolescent.

I don't really get boys. I watch them point sticks at one another and wrestle each other to the ground and think, "Is that fun?" Yet there seems to be a reassuring simplicity to young boys. They aren't sneaky, like I see many girls being. In fact, they're quite obvious about pushing another kid when a toy is taken from them or punching the perpetrator. And from what I hear, boys love their mamas. Who wouldn't want that?

A relationship with a daughter would be much more complicated. At some point, almost all girls have to rebel against their mother. I did, Stacy did, every female friend I have did. It's a given. And again, because of my rape, I may be overprotective of a daughter. I'll freak out as soon as she grows breasts or shows signs of any sexuality, which these days, seems to be as young as eight. It scares me how all girls' clothes are sexy now and pop divas are considered role models. I wore Toughskins and played sports until I was twelve, but I don't know if that's an option for girls nowadays.

The baby is what it is and there's nothing I can do about it. This sounds fatalistic or pessimistic, but really I find it comforting. S/he seems to be happy in my belly, I'm happy having her/him there, I feel good, so why not assume everything is going to be fine? These books want to tell me otherwise, so just like the extra ultrasounds and tests, I think I'll do without them.

ON THE WAY TO OUR NEXT appointment with Afia, I tell Jason, "I'm not so sure about giving birth in a hospital anymore."

"That's so weird, I was just going to say the same thing."

We laugh, knowing this phenomenon all too well. I like to think we're psychically connected, but maybe that's the case for everyone who's lived together for almost nine years.

"It just seems so...."

"Invasive?" I ask.

"Yeah, and I know how you feel about doctors and hospitals. Will you be comfortable there?"

"I doubt it. All the fluorescent lights, nurses bustling in and out, and the monitors constantly beeping at me, it's just not how I imagine giving birth. And the main reason I wanted to be in a hospital was for the drugs, but I don't know if it's worth it just for that. I'd like the chance to at least start somewhere else, to be able to do my own thing, and then if I'm in a ton of pain, I could go get the epidural."

"Can you do that? Or do you have to choose one or the other?"

"Don't know, we can ask Afia."

Afia doesn't seem surprised at all by our announcement that I'm second guessing a hospital birth. When she asks us if we're thinking about a home birth or birth center birth, I say the former and Jason says the latter. So much for our psychic connection.

"From what I understand, a birth center doesn't have any special equipment or staff. It's basically a room that you rent, right?" I ask Afia.

"They have large soaking tubs and birthing balls, but no, they don't have any special medical equipment. Although some are very close to a hospital, so if something went wrong, it would be a simple transfer."

"We live five minutes from a hospital. I'm not worried about that. I like the idea of being able to stay where I am once I'm in labor. I don't want to have to interrupt my rhythm or start over with new people in attendance. That sounds like a nightmare."

"But what about the mess?" Jason asks. "And where would everyone hang out while you're in labor? Our house is too small. The birthing centers probably have rooms for ...."

"Who's 'everyone else'?"

"Our parents and ..."

"I don't know if I want a bunch of people hanging out while I'm in labor. And even if I do, they'd be fine in our house."

As usual, Jason is thinking about other people's feelings. He is a very considerate person. Too considerate, if you ask me. This is about me and my labor, not about our relatives needing more tea to drink while I'm grunting and groaning. Now the mess, that's another story. I considered that as well, remembering the gallons of blood that poured out of Lydia. But Afia quickly alleviates that fear by stating that I could rent a labor tub.

"Water births reduce the strain and pressure on the mother as well as provide a womblike atmosphere for the baby to be born in. The warm water will help regulate your body temperature, which will fluctuate immensely due to all of your exertion, as well as ease your aching muscles. And since the baby is born in the tub, all of the afterbirth goes into the tub, rather than on your carpet."

Sounds good to me. I love water and love the idea of my baby having a gentler transition into this world. No bright lights or cold delivery room, just sliding from one watery womb to another.

My only fear now is the pain. I ask Afia what my options are for pain relief if I deliver at home. She describes several breathing techniques and pressure points, but when I don't look impressed, she says, "I can also bring several herbal remedies."

I was hoping she would be able to offer some real drugs. Herbal remedies are fine when I have a cold, but how helpful are they while giving birth? I want to attempt to go without drugs and like the idea of having to make a conscious decision to ask for them rather than being offered them every five minutes. But I was hoping once I did ask for them, I could immediately have them.

Afia asks me what about labor makes me so nervous. That seems like a silly question to me. Who likes pain? But the more she inquires, the more I understand what she's getting at. Vaginal pain reminds me of being raped; that's why it feels so scary.

"I never describe labor as pain, it's work. And work is hard at times. But what if you start to view it that way as well? As something you're working towards to have your baby and not as something that is being done to you?" she asks.

"OK," I nod. "But, I still think I want drugs."

Afia reassures us again that we don't have to make the decision now; we still have time. She suggests we visit a few birthing centers and tour Swedish hospital's birthing ward so we can get a feel for each place. I feel confident in the information she has given us, agree to think about it more, and believe that, with time, I may be able to let go of the need to have drugs readily available to me.

I'm ready to move on to measuring how big my belly has gotten, but Jason has a few more questions. "What if the baby is breech? What if she hemorrhages? What do you do if there's a prolapsed cord? What if the cord is wrapped around the baby's neck?"

I've seen *The Birth Partner* and even *Worst Case Scenarios: How to Deliver a Baby on Your Own* on his nightstand, but I didn't think he was actually reading them. I'm obviously mistaken. He fires a dozen questions away to Afia, and she calmly answers all of them. I tune most of it out, knowing it is very unlikely that Jason and I will be alone in the woods, miles from civilization, when I go into labor. But when I hear Afia say, "You would stick your hand up her vagina while she keeps her rear in the air as high as possible," I decide to interject. "Enough! You are not going to have to deliver this baby! We live five minutes from a hospital and babies don't shoot out, unfortunately for me."

Jason laughs at the absurdity of it, but I also see him glance down at his notebook. I'm sure he has a few more questions for Afia, but before he can ask them, I say, "Let's listen to the heartbeat."

I'M LEANING TOWARDS A HOMEBIRTH, but the thought of it still scares me. Not only the pain, which is a big concern, but I'm also worried about being safe. I need more information. I know I won't find it in a book, so I start surveying all of the women I know who have given birth.

After several tales of babies born not breathing, or with high fevers, being whisked away and given oxygen, and, the worst story of all, the story of Faith's stillborn baby, I am more confused than ever. All of these scenarios occurred in a hospital, thank goodness, otherwise the mother, baby, or both may not have made it. Even with a team of doctors and medical equipment, no one was able to save Faith's baby. After that harrowing experience, Faith went on to deliver her next baby at home successfully. The cord was wrapped around the baby's neck and he was born blue, but the midwife knew what to do.

This makes me think you can't really know where the safest place is to deliver a baby. Sure, hospitals have lifesaving equipment, but sometimes tragedy occurs and babies die, no matter where you are.

And sometimes it appears that the interventions provided or the changing of the guard is the cause of the problem. A friend of mine gave birth in California. After laboring for twenty four hours, a new doctor came in and said, "Let's get this show on the road." My friend and her doctor had been comfortable allowing the labor to progress along at its slow rate, knowing first time labors are often long, but the new doctor had an agenda. Pitocin was administered, her membranes were stripped, and the contractions started coming at a fierce pace. She could no longer keep up with them or manage the pain, so although she had hoped for an unmedicated birth, she asked for an epidural. Months after her daughter was born, she is still traumatized over the birth. Her birth plan was completely ignored and things escalated to a point where she felt out of control. I don't want this to happen to me, but I also don't want a complication to put my baby or me in danger.

I stop asking women about their labors, it's too nerve wracking, and instead ask them how and why they chose the setting they did. Many women claim they didn't know there was an alternative to a hospital birth, so their decision was easy. Faith's work as a doula and birth advocate made her the perfect homebirth candidate. She didn't seem to ever question that decision, even after her stillbirth years earlier.

The most helpful conversation is with an acupuncturist I have seen off and on for years. She recently delivered her baby at home and when I call Eva to ask her about it, she says, "Before I became pregnant, I liked the idea of having a homebirth, but wasn't sure I would feel comfortable and safe having one. Once I became pregnant, I educated myself about the risks, pros, and cons of a home birth. Intuitively, I knew that's what I wanted, but researching it convinced me. It seems we too often go down the path of fear, of 'what if,' rather than trusting our own strength and ability to go through the pain and exhaustion and come out the other side strong and proud and absolutely ecstatic. I knew I was capable of giving birth on my own, with the help of a midwife, and it seemed the more that women give up that strength and confidence in their bodies, the more likely the birth will end up not being what they wanted."

"You mention comfort and control a few times, which strikes me as funny because I think most people would associate those words with a hospital, yet for you and me, that's what is so enticing about a homebirth," I say.

I want to explore the meaning of those two words with her more, but I hear her baby cry in the background. I thank her for her time and we plan a date to meet for tea and baby ogling.

Her words stick with me all day. I'm doing exactly what she said, going down the "what if" road over and over again, and that's what is preventing me from choosing a homebirth. But what if I were able to go through labor trusting myself and my body and having control over my environment? Not only would I be ecstatic, as Eva said, it would be a giant leap towards feeling proud of my body as a way to heal the damage from the rape.

If I let my fear win, I have to give up comfort. Hospitals make me nervous; I know I won't be comfortable there. And I know I won't be in control either. Sure, Afia will do her best to work with me and keep nurses and anesthesiologists at bay, but it's their turf, not mine. I could easily get swept away.

I can't stand the idea that giving birth could feel similar to being raped. I have to be the one in control of my labor, otherwise I'll feel violated again. I won't let my baby's entrance into this world be a violent act. I want it to feel as safe and nurturing as possible. For both of us.

That night Jason and I meet at Golden Gardens for a picnic. It's a glorious July evening and it will stay light until nearly ten. We spread out a blanket and plop down on it. Kids are racing up and down the beach with their buckets. A stream flows into the Sound and it's the main draw for the kids. They build dams, float sticks down it, and otherwise marvel at the wonder of water.

We watch the kids for a while, both of us imagining what our future child will be like. Will he be the wild freckled boy screaming "All right!" every time his castle survives another wave? Or will she be the little girl in the purple bathing suit, impervious to the cold water?

I take some cheese and crackers out of our cooler and tell Jason about my conversation with Eva. I adopt her calm nature as I relay some of the details of her birth. But when I get to the part about needing control, I feel myself sweat. As if possessed, I suddenly scream out, "It's my fucking body and no one is going to tell me what to do!"

Jason and I sit in silence for a long time. Neither of us are sure what just happened, but we know it was big. Eventually, he looks around to see if any of the kids (or mothers, for that matter) heard my outburst. They seem to be oblivious and he looks relieved.

Tears well up in my eyes as I say, "I need to do this. I need to reclaim my body as mine. I won't let another person have control." I'm thinking of past medical procedures as well as the rape and feel nauseous. Yet, stating these words so adamantly makes me feel strong. Jason starts to lean towards me, changes his mind, and reaches out to hold my hand instead. He's not sure a hug is what I need now and he's right. I've gone back to a world of unjust treatment of my body and am not ready to be held. But holding his hand feels nice. It grounds me and brings me back to the present.

I look at him and say, "I don't want to live in fear." I'm not sure if I'm talking about the rape or my birth fears. It doesn't matter. All that matters is I'm not going to do it anymore.

I KNOW I WANT A HOMEBIRTH, but I'm still nervous about not having any drugs. Jason and I are about to go camping in the Canadian Rockies, so, following Afia's advice, I tell myself I don't need to tackle that issue right now. I still have time.

I fill the car with a queen size air mattress, three pillows, a cooler filled with enough food to feed a small country, and two folding chairs. Jason looks at me skeptically and says, "I thought this camping trip was about simplicity and roughing it?"

"It is." I shove another pillow into the backseat. Jason may need one as well.

"What's with all the stuff then?"

"Roughing it doesn't mean you have to be uncomfortable. I'll feel more serene if I'm full and comfortable."

"Not being able to see out the back window doesn't make me feel serene," he mutters to himself while trying to rearrange and consolidate my goods. I don't have the heart to tell him there's more stuff inside.

Half way across eastern Washington, which is basically a desert, our sunroof sticks. It sticks while open, which is fortunate, because my car's air conditioner hasn't worked for years. I become very nervous when Jason starts fiddling with it, knowing I'm already a little crazy to be camping while seven months pregnant. Not having a sunroof when it's ninety degrees outside could push me over the edge. Just as I'm about to tell him to knock it off, he holds his "tools" (a paperclip and shoelace) up triumphantly and says, "I fixed it!"

Now would be a good time to explain I am no longer a happy drunk. I am a moody drunk, easily irritated and frequently weepy. I also have no control over what I say. Once we cross the Canadian border I repeatedly see signs that say "Litter Barrel Ahead." It becomes the motif for the trip: More shit ahead.

Sometimes I swoon over Jason, and sometimes I cringe when he touches me. I'm not sure if it's due to processing the rape or strictly hormonal, but it's exhausting. It's also confusing. Sometimes I know I'm crying about what was robbed of me as a youth, but other times I have no idea why I'm crying. I just feel incredibly sad. Five minutes later, I'll turn the stereo up, giggle like a school girl, and say, "This is a great trip!" Jason no longer looks at me as if I'm on acid. He just rides the emotional roller coaster with me.

The first couple of times I feel depressed, I try to push it away. I'm on vacation and want to have fun. But I'm learning that the more I accept my feelings, even the negative ones, the quicker they pass. Although I was hoping for a break from thinking about pain, labor, and abuse, this trip offers plenty of opportunities to be still and quiet. And when I'm still, more memories surface. After years of staying busy as a way to avoid my feelings and memories, I'm trying to slow down and let whatever needs to come, come.

I find a grassy patch near the river we're camping by and sit down. As I watch the water turn from an icy blue to a light green, the image of a school gymnasium comes to mind. I'm dancing with an eighth grade boy and he's shoving his hand down my pants and fingering me repeatedly. The details are a little foggy, but my fear and the malicious grin on his face are crystal clear. He's looking at me as if to say, "What are you going to do about it?" I wait for a teacher to rescue me or at least break up our closeness, but they never do. I eventually squirm away and join my friends in the bathroom.

This memory and another of a boy trying to pull my pants down while pushing me into the bushes makes me angry. Not angry with the boys, but angry at myself for not calling out for help or slapping and kicking them. Why did I just stand there and take it? What's wrong with me? Why did I continually let boys treat me so horribly? Why was I so afraid of them?

I know from a book I'm reading about victims of sexual crimes that if the victim tells someone and that person responds appropriately by protecting the victim and only placing blame on the perpetrator, the victim's healing can begin immediately. The longer the secret is held on to and the longer the victim blames herself, the longer the healing will take. I wish I had known this when I was twelve. But the fact is, I was completely ignorant about sex, more so about rape. Nobody explained the birds and bees to me, and whatever was explained to me in health class was out dated and vague. I didn't understand what was happening to me, much less understand that I could scream, fight back, or even tell someone who might've helped me. I went into shock and that's where I've remained for years.

Vicky has taught me that any violation of any orifice is a rape and I need to stop placing my violations in the "not so bad" category. I tend to think women held at knife point are raped and what happened to me doesn't count. But I was raped, at least three times, and acknowledging that is the first step towards learning how to forgive myself.

Although rehashing being raped is awful, I am grateful to have this time to do so. I don't want it to negatively impact my labor or caring for my baby. Not that I believe setting aside a few months is all it's going to take to cure me from being sexually violated, but I am hopeful that it's a good start. Already, I feel progress in recognizing the negative feelings I have about myself. I never knew how much shame, anger, and guilt I had. But now that I do, I can work towards forgiving myself and being proud of my body, not ashamed of it.

A friend who was molested when she was young recently told me, "It's so strange to think that this one event, a ten minute occurrence in my life, years ago, will affect me for my entire life. Not that I haven't had moments of peace, I've had entire years where I didn't think about it a lot, but it's still there, lurking in the background. As my own kids develop, I'll have to work on it again. And sometimes just feeling slighted by a friend can bring up my insecurities all over again."

Rather than feel defeated by her words, as if I'll never heal, I'm trying to view what happened to me as a constant opportunity to learn and grow. Every time I value my body, say no to something I feel is unjust, or stand up for myself, I feel a huge thrill and am immensely proud of myself. Perhaps even more so than if I hadn't been raped. Every time I take care of myself and follow my heart, a little part of me comes alive.

Several months ago, Vicky asked me to take some time to write down all of the things the rape took away from me. And on another piece of paper, she asked me to write all of the things I gained from the rape. "Gained?" I asked incredulously. I was able to fill an entire page of things that were taken from me. My virginity, trust in myself, trust in men, healthy relationships, feeling safe, fear of intimacy, the list went on and on, but the "gained" list was completely blank. Now I have something to put on that page: "opportunity." I am being given the chance to learn how to love and trust myself.

With this new realization, I stand up to go find Jason. My sweet would-never-hurt-a-woman-in-a-million-years-that's-why-I-chose-him husband. When I find him, he can see that I've been crying.

"Are you all right?"

"Yeah," I say. "Want to take a walk with me?"

He says sure and doesn't ask any further questions. It's true that Jason is possibly one of the gentlest men I know, which is wonderful, but it also makes sharing my hardship with him difficult. I see how appalled, hurt, and confused he becomes when hearing stories about my adolescence. He honestly can't believe such a thing would happen. Not that he thinks I'm lying, but part of him would like to believe I'm exaggerating or don't have the details straight so he can continue to believe the world is a safe place. So I keep a lot of it to myself.

AFTER "ROUGHING IT" for several days, I want to spoil myself by going to one of the hot springs in the Canadian Rockies. I can hardly control my enthusiasm as I strip off my clothes and get ready to submerge myself in the soothing water. Just as I'm about to do so, an ominous black and white sign warning pregnant women not to use the hot springs catches my eye. "Damn it," I mutter to myself. I weigh my desire over my fear for the baby and hope that Jason doesn't notice the sign. He's the rule follower in the family, and I know what he'll say about the matter. But I also know he's not the one with the aching back and restless legs. Nor is he the one carrying an extra thirty pounds of baby making material around. If I only submerge myself half way in the water and am careful not to become overheated, I'm sure the baby will be fine.

One foot into the water and I know I've made the right choice. By the time I'm waist deep, all I can say is, "Ahhhh."

My relief is interrupted when Jason says, "Hey, look at that sign." I tell him my rationale, but his brow remains furrowed.

"Come on, honey. It's not that big of a deal. I've been so good for the whole pregnancy. I've barely had any alcohol, I go for a walk every day, take my vitamins and go to prenatal yoga every week. One little stint in a hot spring won't do any harm. It feels so good, I don't want to get out yet."

"Well, I can't tell you what to do, but…"

"You're right, you can't. So, let me have this, OK? I promise not to get overheated. If I feel flushed or dizzy, I'll immediately get out."

"OK," he sighs.

I can't help giggling about our conversation. Before I was pregnant, I never claimed I would do all of this. I didn't plan on getting drunk every weekend, but I didn't think I'd abstain from alcohol altogether either. I figured I'd have a glass of wine when I felt like it and not worry about it too much. It ends up that I rarely feel like drinking, so have pretty much abstained completely.

The first time I walked into my prenatal yoga class and heard all of those women talking about perineums and cervixes, I almost turned around and left. And when I saw all of those large women squatting, I thought, "Yeah right. That will never be me." Not only did I have a hard time imagining I would ever be that big, I was also damned sure I wouldn't be crouching and squatting while in my third trimester.

Seven months later, I'm a yoga groupie. I never miss my class, have a somewhat unhealthy obsession with my teacher Ellen, and am furious whenever there's a sub. I'm the first to bring up perineums and fear of hemorrhoids, and I may not be the largest person in the class yet, but once I am, I know I'll be front and center squatting and stretching as best as I can.

"I can't believe how good this feels," Jason says. The furrow is gone, which means he is no longer worried about our unborn baby. That's a relief. Too much of a good thing can be overkill. Sure, I want to do what's right for my baby, but I have to indulge myself every once in a while too.

"It's amazing, isn't it? My back doesn't hurt anymore and my whole body feels like spaghetti. I'm really glad we came."

"Hmmm," is all he says. His eyes are closed and he has a smile on his face.

I wonder if the labor pool will be as soothing as these hot springs. Afia said they're six feet in diameter and I'll be able to fit my whole body inside. If that's the case, maybe it will ease my pain. Or at least dull it significantly. I think about it more, remind myself that the pain of birth is working towards something, not taking something away from me, and then announce to Jason, "I don't need drugs. I want to try to deliver the baby at home."

"I know, but we're going to check out the birth centers and hospital before we decide. Right?"

"No, I don't need to see those places. If the labor tub is anything like this hot spring, I'll be happy. And if it's not, well, we'll have to deal with that then." I'm trying to sound cavalier, but Jason knows how afraid I am of the pain.

"I need to do this. I can't really explain why, but I really need to birth my baby at home. Or at least try to. If I can't, I can't. But I need to at least try to trust myself. My body has known what to do so far, I think it will know what to do during labor. Right?"

"I don't know, it's not for me to say. It feels like your thing. Something you need to do for yourself."

"It is."

"You know I'll support you in whatever you choose."

'Thanks," I smile. "I'm taking something back. Something that never should have been taken away in the first place."

We hold each other's gaze for a minute, but don't talk. Eventually, he says, "So, it's decided then?"

"Yup. I'm not going to second guess myself or my body anymore. I can do this, I can try to birth my baby at home."

WITHIN FIVE MINUTES of returning to Seattle, I want to run back to Canada. The answering machine is full of people asking about syllabi, the status of articles, and baby shower ideas. I am not ready to deal with any of these topics. I flip through the mail, but even that disgruntles me. I think about checking my emails when the phone rings. I answer it tentatively and am relieved when I hear Jennifer's voice.

"We're going swimming in Lincoln Park."

I start to protest, but she says, "Come on, you can always nap later. I'm picking you up in fifteen minutes. Pack a towel, your suit, and some sunblock. I'll bring everything else. Including food."

You would think I would resent being bossed around so much, but actually I love it. I'm incapable of thinking straight these days, so direct orders are greatly appreciated.

I've been spending a lot of time in my backyard plastic swimming pool, but it's no comparison to the huge outdoor, heated, saltwater pool that overlooks the Sound and Vashon Island. Lincoln Park is on the western tip of West Seattle, and its pool is surrounded by the beach. The only way you could be closer to the Sound was if you were swimming in it. But I'll take a heated pool over the 55 degree Sound any day. Submerging my body in the salt water feels great. Jennifer swims, but all I can do is bob around.

The temperature drops, my hands prune up, and I decide I've had enough bobbing for one day. While showering, I notice three little girls watching me. They stare at my belly, breasts, back to my belly, and then look at my face. I act as if I don't notice them staring, but every once in a while, we catch each other's eyes. I look away immediately, but they keep staring unabashedly. Once they have fully absorbed my body, they move on to their own bodies. They rub themselves with joy and play in the water.

I can't bring myself to rub my vagina with glee like the little girls do, but with them as my role models, I walk around the locker room naked without feeling self conscious. I even get a few long looks at other women's bodies and marvel at the differences. Almost everyone is staring at my giant belly. Seeing as I don't mind, I assume they feel the same way. Otherwise, we wouldn't be parading around naked.

I return home proud, rejuvenated, and famished. Jason returns shortly after me with burritos in hand. I swoon with love, for him and the food. While I'm stuffing my face with sour cream, beans, and cheese, he says, "My mom called and she wants to know what you want for the baby."

"I already told her we're good."

"Yeah, she seems to think we need a few things. She said she'd take you shopping for a crib, swing, high chair, clothes for the baby, a monitor…"

"I hate to shop. We don't need any of that stuff."

"I'm starting to think we might need some of it. If you don't want to buy it yourself, let people buy it for you at the shower."

"I don't want the stupid shower and I don't give a fuck what people buy me! What I really want is a year's supply of diapers, but no one wants to get me that so they can go ahead and fill our house with crap for all I care."

"They're just trying to help." Jason is used to my outbursts these days, but that doesn't prevent him from taking a step away from the table and looking at me as if I'm a wild animal about to spring from her cage. Which is pretty close to how I feel.

I know people are just being nice, but I really don't want a shower. I don't mind the party part, it's the gift part that throws me. I'm not one to get excited over unnecessary frivolities and I hate opening gifts in front of people.

"I know how you feel about 'things,' but a few items could be really helpful. Like a stroller and some clothes," Jason cautions.

"Diane's given me a ton of stuff."

I smile at the memory of my friend hauling three garbage bags out of her car while saying, "Here's a bunch of Gabe's clothes. I washed all of the buggers and barf off, but don't feel as if you have to keep any of this crap. I just want to get rid of it." That's the kind of gift giving I like. Recycled clothes with no pretenses.

"Yeah, but we might need more."

"All right," I mutter. "I'll think about it."

While washing the dishes I realize my agitation is due to feeling as if I'm not doing enough for my baby. I felt the same way the day I ran into a friend of Faith's, a midwife who asked about a belly cast, five million different herbs and vitamins she assumed I was taking, and the pregnancy photos and rituals she was sure I had completed by now. I mumbled a few excuses and ran away from her. All the way home I chided myself. "I'm too cheap to take care of my baby's nutrition. I'm too lazy to get a belly cast. I'm a horrible person."

When I recall the situation now, I realize Faith's friend was being intrusive. She didn't even know me, yet felt perfectly comfortable telling me what to do. As Vicky pointed out, rather than being angry at her, I was angry at myself. And now, having people offer to buy stuff for my baby makes me feel guilty and angry again. As if I'm already failing as a mother.

"That's bullshit," I say. I stop washing the dishes and look for more plates to smash. Looks as if we're running low, I'll have to use rocks. I stomp outside and start hurling rocks at the trashcan. God, it feels good to let go of my anger. With every throw of a rock, I tell myself I am doing enough. I am good.

"Hey, it's your mom on the phone. Want me to take a message?" Jason calls out the door. After he lamented the loss of his favorite coffee cup, he's become supportive of my rock throwing, plate smashing routine. He even offered to find me a punching bag that we could hang from the basement ceiling, but I said the rocks were satisfying me for now.

After two more throws, I brush off my hands and take the phone from Jason. "Hi, Mom."

"Hey. I want to plan a special day with you so we can have some sacred time."

I look at the phone in disbelief. This can't be my mother. But why would someone impersonate her? My mom never uses words such as sacred. In fact, she rarely even calls me. "What did you have in mind?" I ask.

"I thought we could go shopping for the baby."

Shopping is sacred? Hardly. But this does reassure me that it actually is my mother on the phone. I had no idea that the grandmothers were so worried about my inadequately stocked nursery.

I remind myself it's my nursery they think is inadequate, not me, and agree to the sacred day. I know buying things for my baby has no impact on my mothering skills. I will be a good mother even if my baby has to wear clothes with stains on them. I also know I can say no to anything that seems unnecessary and only accept what might be helpful. I have choices. I can say no and be heard.

AFTER SITTING AROUND in my pajamas for two hours eating, drinking decaf, and chatting with my mom on the front porch, I have to agree, this is sacred time. The sun is out, the garden is in full bloom, and we've done nothing but eat and talk. I couldn't have planned a more special day.

But now she wants to take me stroller shopping. I can't imagine anything worse than stepping foot into a mega-baby store, but I know my mom really wants to do this for me and I'll get a free stroller out of it. Something I actually do want. I root around Jason's closet for his last pair of shorts that still fit me. When I can't button them, I add maternity clothes to the shopping list.

I know I want a jogging stroller, but the store we're in only has one model, so I turn around to leave. I look back and see that instead of following me, my mom has a pen and notebook in her hand and is writing copious notes about God only knows what.

"What are you doing?"

"I like to compare the different models and their features…"

I cut her off mid-sentence and say, "When I see they don't have what I want, I get the hell out of the store."

She says that's fair enough and we move on. After what feels like hours, we return home with three maternity bras and a book shelf. Somehow, I don't think these things are going to help my baby, but I'm proud to have bought things I wanted, rather than what someone else wanted for me.

My mom rests in the shade while I sit in my haven, the plastic swimming pool. We're supposed to meet my father for dinner soon, but we both need some time to recover from the fluorescent lights and hundreds of people swarming the hellish Babies "R" Us. I make a vow right then to never, ever step foot in that store again.

My dad arrives about an hour later to find my mom and me chatting in the shade of our maple tree. I hug him hello and he pulls up a chair to join us. Within a few minutes of small talk, the conversation turns to my pregnancy.

"Which hospital are you going to deliver in?" my dad asks nonchalantly.

I see Jason about to walk out to our deck, drinks in hand, but upon hearing that question, he sneaks back inside. Smart move. We haven't told any family members about our home birth decision yet. Based on the "Why would you do that?" reactions I've received upon telling a few acquaintances, I've become reluctant to talk about it.

People seem to think that opting for a homebirth is analogous to a death wish. A friend of Jason's even regaled him with a horror story about how his sister nearly bled to death when she birthed her child at home. Jason returned home pale and second guessing our decision. I calmed him down by mentioning that maybe his friend was exaggerating, seeing as I know his sister lived to have another baby at home, and that she also lives in a very rural area, which we don't.

I cautiously tell my dad, "I'm going to have a home birth."

"What the hell does that mean?"

"I wouldn't be in a hospital, unless I have to transfer there. I'd deliver the baby at home with Afia."

"What? You're shitting me! No goddamn way! I can't believe you. You want to do everything at home. You work here, got married here, and now want to have your baby here? Unfuckingbelievable!"

My dad stomps around the deck, lights three cigarettes in a row, and mutters more profanities while I laugh to myself. I'm used to my father's tirades, and I know this will blow over in a matter of minutes. What I find funny is, he's right. I do want to do everything at home.

He looks to my mother for support, but she merely shrugs. They rarely meddle in my life, so I expect the same today. My dad has tried to influence me a few times, like when he asked me if I was going to go to Princeton or Cornell when it came time to apply for colleges. I laughed and said, "Neither! I'm done jumping through hoops to get As. I want to relax and study what I feel like. You can't do that at those schools, they're too intense." My dad wasn't pleased, but he let the subject drop quickly and even toured several liberal arts colleges with me. When I dropped out of my non-Ivy League college to travel and "experience real life for awhile," my father panicked that I would get knocked up and never return to school. He never said as much to me, but my mom told me years later. They may not always approve of my decisions, but they never forbid them. And I suspect the same about my choice to deliver the baby at home. Even if they oppose it, they'll resign themselves to it.

"Dr. Jack is rolling over in his grave," my dad mutters. Dr. Jack being my mother's father, an Ob-Gyn.

I look at my mom to see if this is going to raise any hackles. She worships her father and he seemed to be somewhat of a hero before he died. If anything is going to get a reaction, this will. But she merely smiles and turns her attention back to her magazine.

After a few more stomps and choice swear words, my father sits back down. "So you're dead set on this?"

"Yeah."

"And it's safe?"

"Yes. Afia has delivered numerous babies at home, all without complications."

"If something goes wrong, you'll go to a hospital, right?"

"Absolutely. And it's only a short drive away. Or we'll call an ambulance."

He takes a large drag off of his cigarette and nods his head. "Where are we eating tonight?"

And that is the end of the homebirth discussion with my parents.

AFTER MY PARENTS' RELATIVELY subdued reaction to hearing I'm planning on a homebirth, we feel ready to tell Jason's parents as well. Compared to my father, Jason's parents are extremely mellow and quiet. I can't think of a time that I've ever seen any of his parents yell, or even raise their voice for that matter. They've never told us we're making a poor choice or criticized us. We don't see them that often and when we do, the visits are usually quite pleasant and always cordial.

First, we drive to Bellingham to tell his mother. I try to read her expression, but it's difficult. She smiles politely and asks a few "is that safe?" questions. I've learned that everyone relaxes once they hear how close we live to a hospital and that I am not opposed to transferring there if I need to. "We live five minutes from the hospital," has become my mantra. I see some of the concern leave her face once she hears this and the discussion ends shortly thereafter.

Once we finish lunch with his mother, we drive to Samish Island to tell his father and stepmom. They both nod their head and say, "Interesting." Jason's father, always the history teacher, starts to recite several tribal birthing practices and Eileen, a librarian, fills in with several anecdotes of her own. After hearing about the strength of Amazon women and tales of women squatting in the fields, barely pausing their harvesting to birth a baby, I interject, "I'm not actually planning on delivering the baby outside. We're going to rent a labor tub and deliver the baby in that." This seems to pique their interest and they become rather animated about the "one watery womb to another" metaphor.

"That sounds wonderful," Eileen says. "What a peaceful way to come into the world."

We hope so, I think to myself.

Stacy is not nearly as excited about the watery womb idea. "So, you'll be sitting in this big tub with all of your own blood and guts? Like a big stew? Gross."

"Better that than to have it spill all over my carpet."

"Why would you want to do that? Don't you want as many nurses and doctors present as possible?"

"No, I actually want as few people as possible there."

"Not me. If I ever have a baby, I'm going to have everyone I know in the hospital room with me. It will be a huge party."

The image of a party like atmosphere at my birth is as shocking and repulsive to me as the idea of a homebirth stew is to Stacy. Revelry, noise, chatter, and chaos are things that Stacy adores, but for me, that would be a nightmare. I want it to be quiet, calm, and peaceful and I want the focus to be on the baby, not having a good time or catching up with old acquaintances.

The people in my everyday life, friends and the women from the paper, seem to view birthing a child at home as completely normal. Even if they didn't or wouldn't choose to do so themselves, they understand my desire to do so. By working at home and rarely going out or meeting new people, my world has become rather small. And in this world, it is normal to talk about labor tubs and dilation. But every once in a while, that bubble is burst, such as when a woman from my yoga class says she is hoping for an early elective C-section because her doctor will be traveling during her due date. Or when my aunt calls me and scolds me for wanting a home birth. "Just wait until your uncle hears this," she says. "He's going to have some things to say."

Of all my relatives, my sixties-loving, lived-in-a-yurt, boyfriend-dodged-the-draft aunt is the last person I thought would disapprove of my birth choice. I idolized her as a child and even chose to go to college in the town where she and my uncle live. I loved spending weekends with them, listening to all their old records, digging through her closet for beaded shirts and bell bottom jeans, and eating tofu and curry with them, delicacies never served in my own home. I feel betrayed that this role model of freedom and anti-establishment is not supporting my decision. But after she warns me about hemorrhaging and complications, I start to understand why she is so concerned. She once helped a friend give birth at home and there were problems. My aunt lives in rural, upstate New York and the nearest hospital is a half an hour away. This experience convinced her that home births are dangerous. I reassure her that we're in a metropolitan area and can receive help within a matter of minutes.

"I still don't like the idea and think you should reconsider," she says and then hands the phone to my uncle. My uncle was a hippie as well, also lived in a yurt, and built the house he and my aunt currently live in, but he now works in a hospital as an administrator. He is a gentle, soft spoken man and I've always felt very close to him, but I know his work at the hospital may cause him to feel apprehensive about my decision. I brace myself for more birth horror stories, but instead he asks about Afia.

"So, you say she's a midwife and a naturopath? Is that like an osteopath?"

"No, she's not an MD, she's an ND. Naturopaths consider the whole body and the mind as well when diagnosing problems."

"Interesting, I've never heard of that. How close is the nearest hospital?"

"Five minutes."

"And you'll be careful? Get help if you need it?"

"Of course."

"All right then, good luck."

Not exactly the "choice words" I was warned about and a much better conversation than I expected. And after this conversation, I try to remember to think twice before speaking. If I'm in the company of close friends or the women from the paper, I can feel free to discuss water births and midwives. In any other company, it's best to keep quiet. If I fail to remember this, which is inevitable, I'll pull out my mantra as quickly as possible. "I only live five minutes from the hospital."

ALTHOUGH I'M ENJOYING spending most of the summer gardening and lounging around in my inflatable swimming pool, I'm thrilled when it's time to start working on the October issue of *Women of Seattle*. I've missed working. I gain a lot of satisfaction from talking with other writers. I love reading their stories and having the "aha" moment when I understand what's missing or seeing how the story could be improved. And I love discussing the changes with the authors and how it connects us, as if we are creating something together.

I'm trying to follow my own advice and have started reshaping and revising several of my journal entries. Most of them are stream of consciousness, or, more recently, rants. Besides throwing rocks, I'm expressing my anger on paper and writing letters that I'll never send to people who have hurt me. Amongst the therapeutic but disjointed rants are a few pearls. By adding context and sharpening details, I'm able to see a clear story emerge. Once I have two or three complete, I start looking for publications to send them to.

After selecting a few publications with a similar voice as mine, I start to doubt the quality of my writing. I tell myself my articles aren't good enough to be published, and that I'm kidding myself that I can actually write something someone else would be interested in reading. I can't stand the idea of being rejected, because it would not only be an insult to my writing, but would insult me as a person as a well.

I know this is irrational. Vicky's words, "You are your own worst critic. You are a strong, powerful, intelligent woman. Can't you see that?" run through my mind. I believe her, when I'm sitting across from her, but not when I'm composing an email to an editor.

I try to push myself to send the articles anyway, but when my stomach tightens, I stop. I have to listen to my gut and it's telling me I'm not ready yet. Maybe I'll try again in a few months.

Later that day, I laugh at the absurdity of the situation. Here I am, the editor of a publication for women, full of personal essays, yet I'm trying to connect with large publications three thousand miles away. When I think about writing for *Women of Seattle*, I feel excited, not terrified. I ask the Council if I can submit an essay about my miscarriage and am met with a resounding, "Yes! We were wondering when you were going to write something."

Writing about the loss, fear, and deep despair that I felt last winter feels so incongruous with sitting here now, the sun pouring through the window onto my huge belly. Although I am so grateful to feel as if I have everything that I want, I don't want to ever forget Sweet Pea. I walk out to my front yard to visit the hosta Jason and I planted as a tribute to Sweet Pea.

As I water the hosta and pick off a few snails, an excerpt from the book I'm reading, *Catching Babies*, comes to mind. A young boy tells his mother, who had just miscarried, that the miscarried baby returns to heaven and waits its turn to be born again. I'm not sure I believe in heaven, but I have always found comfort in believing there is something else after we die, maybe reincarnation or a tranquil holding place, such as the boy in the book described. I like believing that perhaps I'll be able to meet Sweat Pea.

Sweat begins to trickle down between my breasts and down my forehead, so I say good-bye to Sweet Pea and get out of the sun. The front of my house receives unfiltered sunlight from early morning until almost noon. This is glorious ninety percent of the time, but this August we're having a stretch of ninety-degree days, which is considered unbearably hot. Most Seattle homes, including mine, don't have air conditioning, so we rely on the ever present breeze coming off the Sound and fans to cool our homes. All this said, I'm still sweating like a pig, even indoors.

Jason's shorts no longer fit, so I've moved on to two muumuus that a friend passed on to me. At least they keep me relatively cool. My wardrobe choices these days are limited to muumuus or extra large boxer shorts that I bought at Fred Meyer. It's a good thing I rarely leave the house.

I've somehow convinced myself that since I'm pregnant and work from home, I no longer have to look acceptable. I pretend that on the rare occasions I do leave, it's all right that I'm wearing boxer shorts with frogs on them or a flowered muumuu because no one notices me. I think no one is paying attention to the crazy pregnant frog lady and even if they are, they'll excuse me for being crazy (or abrupt, or loud, or unhygienic, or forgetful, or lazy) because I'm pregnant. I guess I'm still pretending I'm invisible.

My belly is larger than my breasts, so men no longer leer at me. Now they smile compassionately, or look away nervously. Either way, I feel protected by my pregnancy. My body is no longer viewed as a sexual item, so I don't have to fear being violated. It's as if I went from whore to Madonna over night, which is strange because I wouldn't be pregnant if I didn't have sex. My sexuality is more apparent now than any other time in my life, yet it's being negated. I find comfort in this. All men see is my pregnancy and, ironically, no longer deem me as a sexual person to leer at.

When I do leave the house, almost always in search of food, I'm drawn to other misfits wearing frogs and muumuus. I frequently strike up conversations with vendors of *Real Change*, Seattle's homeless persons newspaper, and have made quite a few connections with elderly people. At the grocery store, I'll groan with an octogenarian about why so many of the items we need are either on the bottom or top shelf. Stooping down is painful enough, but trying to rise again from a crouch is near impossible. As for jumping up to reach an item, that's never going to happen.

Although I feel camaraderie with the older generation, I do notice that our ways of dealing with these difficulties vary considerably. After trying to quickly cross the street, seeing as the car heading towards us is not slowing down—in fact, it appears that it is speeding up—my elderly companion smiles sweetly and says, "My, my. Everyone is in such a hurry these days." My response is to give the driver the finger and say, "That crazy asshole almost tried to kill us. I know he saw us, how could he not with this bull's-eye of a belly, yet he didn't even slow down. What a jerk." While they wait patiently for someone to get their favorite strawberry jelly from the top shelf, I stand on a lower shelf, nearly breaking it and possibly my ankle as well, and curse the store and all of its employees for making access to sugar so difficult. We may both be wearing muumuus, and neither of us can move quickly anymore, but the similarities stop there.

V
Third Trimester
Fall

Third Trimester-Fall

ALTHOUGH I EAGERLY AGREED to teach three classes in the fall and nearly begged to get my teaching job back, now that school is actually going to start, I'm second guessing my decision. OK, that's an understatement. I'm horrified. First of all, I'll have to leave the house on a weekly basis. Second of all, I'll actually have to shower and wear something besides my muumuu on some of these occasions. Third of all, I'll have to talk to other people in a somewhat coherent fashion. Fourth of all, these "other people" will be middle-schoolers.

Just as I'm about to call the director to see if she can replace me, I remember my bank account. I tell myself I'm lucky to have work at all and drag myself out of bed. But by day four, I know I made the wrong choice. Not only is teaching proving to be difficult, I made the wrong choice in students. When deciding between returning to my adult writing classes or the classes for kids, I chose the kids, thinking they would be more fun to be around while eight months pregnant. I couldn't be more wrong.

A large percentage of the kids spent the majority of their summer "hangin' out playing vids and watching tv." Not only do I have a huge bias against television and video games, and the rotting of the brain I am sure they contribute to, but I'm also appalled that these kids spent so much time inside. What about exercise and fresh air? What about the beach, copious parks, and forests that are all nearby? Aren't summers meant to be spent outside?

Whenever I ask the kids to answer a simple question or critically examine something, "Huh?" is all they can muster. They appear to be bewildered by the fat lady who keeps talking to them. I can almost see them searching for the remote control.

One girl spends half of class putting on eye shadow. I am about to ask her to stop, but then remember how whenever she speaks, I can't decipher what she's saying through all of the "likes," "ums," and giggles. I pretend not to notice when she splays six lip glosses out on her desk. At least that will keep her quiet.

Without intending to be, I am once again surrounded by thirteen-year-old boys. Perhaps subconsciously I chose my kid classes over the adult classes as a way to test myself. To see if I would feel uncomfortable and need to race home and take a shower after every class or if I would avoid eye contact with the boys and mainly focus on the girls. For the most part, this is not the case. There are two boys in my class that I feel nervous around. They already have facial hair, cocky grins, and a swagger when they walk. They feel like men compared to the other boys in my class who still speak with high voices, would rather play computer games than talk to girls, and are completely awkward in their bodies. When addressing the "older" boys, my palms sweat and I notice I stammer more. So far, reminding myself that I'm safe, that this is now and that was then, seems to be enough.

But when I see the boys flirt with girls, I feel nauseous. I tell myself that it would be inappropriate for me to run over to the girl and grab her in my arms to protect her, even though that is what I want to do. I can't protect every adolescent girl, but I can hope that I have some influence in my students' lives. I hope that my class encourages them to think for themselves, assert their ideas and needs, and critically examine situations. I can listen to them and hopefully offer guidance, but I can't protect all of them.

By the third week, the majority of the kids seem to have the use of their brains back. They are able to write and speak coherently and are even witty and intelligent at times. I wish I could say the same for myself. I can remain somewhat articulate and patient through my first and second classes, but I'm pretty much a raving lunatic by the third one. The kids don't even bat an eye during most of my outbursts and ramblings. They're all high on hormones as well, they understand.

And the women on the Wisdom Council have either been pregnant, are experiencing menopause, or at least have had their bouts with PMS. Hormones are no stranger to these women. Thank God, otherwise they would have kicked me out months ago.

While sitting in a production meeting, discussing something arbitrary, such as the state of the world, Faith notices I'm being unusually quiet.

"Corbin, what do you think about the war in Iraq?" she asks.

"I don't know, I stopped paying attention about seven months ago. But I do know I'm starving. How much longer is this going to take?"

The pregnancy Get Out of Jail for Free card is still working for me. Instead of thinking I'm rude, which I am, Faith and another woman jump up to make me a sandwich.

Once I'm satisfied with the ample amount of food I'm served, I can focus on the details of production. We discuss the new layout and I tell everyone about the articles I have so far. One of the columnists wrote about being single and her dating life. I get so carried away relaying her story that I don't realize I'm now sharing my own sexual stories.

"My friend gave me a dildo a few months back and I've already been through a set of batteries. Jason acts insulted when I pull the vibrator out and says, 'I'm right here!'

"'I know,' I say, 'but you have to go to work. Close the door when you leave, OK? And take the cat with you.'"

Some of the women laugh, but several look embarrassed. How did I get from page layout to dildos? And why am I telling these women about it?

Appropriate and inappropriate conversation has become blurry for me. I'm so proud that I actually use the vibrator, rather than let it gather dust, which is what I assumed it would do, I want to share my triumph. I've leaped over a huge hurdle to be able to masturbate freely and touch myself "down there." Giving myself pleasure and exploring my labia and clitoris rather than pretending they don't exist is a milestone for me. But perhaps not one to share at the work place.

I'M SITTING ON THE COUCH talking to my baby as I push against his/her bum. S/he rolls and I feel a foot. I push against that and feel another roll. I've been playing this game a lot and although I find it fascinating to be able to decipher a head, butt, and foot, I'm not sure I should spend the next six weeks doing this. I'd love to, but there are probably more important things to take care of.

Such as finding a doula. Eight months ago, I didn't even know what a doula was, but Faith's stories about her work as a doula intrigue me. She describes it as having someone at the birth to focus on the laboring mother. I assumed that's what Afia and her assistant would be doing, but Faith clarifies the different roles for me. "Of course Afia is going to help you, but she's also concentrating on the baby. She's a medical professional, so she has to monitor the birth as a whole and make sure it's progressing normally. A doula's main concern is you and how she can help you."

When I overhear Ellen, my favorite prenatal yoga instructor, tell someone she is a doula, as well as a massage therapist, I'm sold on the idea of a doula. I feel comfortable with Ellen, know how much she's helped me in yoga class, and feel confident that her training as a doula, as well as her own experiences giving birth four times, offer her more knowledge and expertise than Jason or I have.

Ellen comes over to our house to meet with Jason and me. Similar to our meeting with Afia, I instantly know this is the doula for me. I look at Jason and he nods. When Ellen asks us if we'd like some time to think it over, I say, "No. If you're available, I'd love to have you at my birth."

I set up a meeting for the following week so Ellen can meet Afia and Lisa, Afia's assistant. I'm confident in my team and don't have any doubts that they are going to fully support me, yet something is still nagging at me. Something feels unsettled.

I think it's my lack of gear for the baby. I make a list of "recommended items" and plan on going shopping after my appointment with Vicky. I explain the unsettled feeling I have to her and she says, "And you think it's about not having enough stuff for the baby?"

"Maybe. Isn't that what new mothers do? Buy a bunch of stuff?"

"But is that what you need?"

It doesn't take long to realize that is not my problem. The baby will sleep with us at first and I have plenty of clothes for him/her. I'm just trying to busy myself again.

"Are you worried about the birth?" Vicky asks.

"A little."

"Do you want me to walk you through some more guided visualizations?"

"No."

"Did you pick some items to hold on to, to ground you?"

"Yeah, a rose quartz crystal and my favorite river rock."

"But you need something else."

"I think so, but I don't know what."

"Your gut knows." Vicky hands me a piece of paper. "Let your intuition tell you what you need."

With my right hand I write, "What do you need at the birth?" I place the pen in my left hand, and without thinking about it write, "Listen to me."

Almost every time I do this exercise I'm shocked at what my left hand writes. It appears to come out of nowhere, yet every time it taps into something core. I brush away my tears and look up at Vicky. "I'm not sure why I'm crying."

"When you were raped, you weren't listened to. I think the little girl inside of you wants to make sure that doesn't happen again."

My body slumps with relief. That's it. That's what I need: to be heard. I've spent all of this time and energy making sure I have the ideal birth scenario, that all of the people present will listen to me and understand my wishes, yet the person I really fear won't listen to me is me. I'm afraid I'll emotionally shut down or ignore my instincts and let fear take over, or only listen to my critical self.

Although I'm crying even harder now, the agitated feeling is gone. I don't need baby gear, I need to learn how to trust myself.

Vicky says, "You have a very strong intuition and it will help you during labor if you can trust it. Do you think you can do that?"

"I think so."

"Let's shoot for a solid 'yes' before this baby comes," she says.

I STILL END UP HAVING TO GO shopping. But rather than onesies and bouncy chairs, I buy the birth supplies from Afia's list.

I dump a mountain of receiving blankets, a spray bottle, maxi pads, witch hazel, gel ice packs, large disposable pads, baby syringes, and an extra shower curtain to protect our sheets on the floor of our guest room. I imagine the labor tub being set up in the corner, the sheets and towels that will be spread over the carpet, and me crouching on the floor grunting. I feel excited rather than scared and tell myself, "I'm ready."

I pull my tarot cards out and start to do a reading about the birth. I stop myself before I flip the first card over. I don't want to look to the cards for my fate, I can rely on myself for that. I have to trust that no matter what happens, I'll know what the right thing to do is. I have to listen to myself, not the cards.

Jason comes upstairs and finds me leaning against the wall in the guest room, smugly rubbing my belly. "I'm ready," I say.

"Cool, because Stacy just called with the details."

"Huh?" *Details of my labor*, I think. *How the hell does she have those?*

He laughs. "She knew you were going to say that and even said, 'Don't pretend like you forgot about the shower and don't try to get out of it because Mom and I already planned the menu.'"

"Didn't she want to talk to me?"

"No, she was headed out. She just wanted to make sure you'd be there."

I go downstairs and debate who to call first. I decide on my mom.

"Mom, I told you I wasn't sure I wanted a shower."

"I know you did, but I decided we needed to have one anyway. It's the first grandchild. It's a big deal."

"You're really not going to let me get out of this?"

"No."

I'm so shocked, I have to get off the phone. My mother never makes me do things I don't want to do. Not only did she subject me to the horrors of Babies "R" Us, but now she's making me have a party. What's gotten into her?

"What's up with Mom?" I ask Stacy as soon as she answers her cell phone.

"What do you mean?"

"Why is she so into the shower idea?"

"A better question is why are you so against it? Parties are fun. You should be glad we're throwing you one. Anytime you feel like buying a bunch of food for me and pouring me a glass of champagne, I'm game."

I hang up with Stacy, feeling ashamed. It's incredibly generous of my mom to open up her house to all of my friends. And it's wonderful the way she and Stacy are trying to take care of me and support the baby. I know they will spend a lot of time cooking and buying delicious food. What's so bad about that?

I place a third and final call to my friend Jennifer. After explaining the situation to her, she says, "It's because you don't like being the center of attention."

I'm about to protest, then realize she's right.

"And you have a thing against stuff. The whole point of a baby shower is to get stuff and fawn all over the mother-to-be. It's your biggest nightmare."

"But my mom really wants to have it for me. What do I do?"

"When it comes time to open the gifts, let everyone open one for you. Most people love presents, so they'll be excited to help you. It takes the pressure off of you and gets you out of the spotlight."

"You're a genius!"

I hang up with Jennifer and for the first time actually start to look forward to the shower. When friends call to ask me what I want, I tell them books. "Hard, cardboard books that the baby can chew on." If they sound less than excited about the book idea, I say, "Or you can get the baby some clothes. Something practical though, OK?"

When I arrive at the shower, I see my mom and Stacy have been hard at work. They've enlisted the help of my aunt and cousin, who are visiting from New York, and they have formed a well-oiled catering team.

"Would you like a glass of orange juice, champagne, or a combination of both?" my cousin asks.

"Both." I'm giddy with the anticipation of my first drink in months. Being surrounded by all of my friends and family on a glorious, sunny October day is definitely a call for celebration.

I'm offered mimosas all day long, but never seem to actually get to drink one. I'll have one sip and then place it down to hug a friend or go to the bathroom and when I look around for it, it's gone. The well-oiled catering team may be taking their roles too seriously.

We all sit on my mom's deck and enjoy the unexpected, warm day. Stacy made a veggie lasagna, my mom made several quiches, my aunt is cutting up a huge bowl of fruit, there's an impressive smoked salmon platter, and there are lots and lots of desserts. I get so carried away with chatting, and eating four platefuls of food, that I forget that I didn't want to have this party.

Even opening presents isn't as heinous as I thought it would be. Jennifer's plan works out wonderfully and everyone dives into the gifts. I watch Stacy lift a beautiful sweater off of the mound of board books. She fingers the delicate scalloped edge, rubs the incredibly soft knit against her face, and sighs, "It's gorgeous."

I contemplate giving her the sweater, knowing my baby will probably only puke on it, so why not let someone have it who will appreciate it? But then I remember Stacy doesn't want a baby, so why would she want a baby sweater?

Before I know it, everyone is hugging me good-bye. I help clean up and then sit on the couch with Stacy. I have a huge piece of lemon tart in one hand and the much anticipated mimosa in the other. What a luxury.

"That wasn't too bad," Stacy says.

"That's what I was going to say. You're the party person, why would that have been bad for you?"

"Because I thought everyone would ask me when I'm going to have a baby. Or even worse, ask when I'm going to get married. But only two people asked, so I consider that a success."

I never thought about how it could be awkward for Stacy, seeing as she is the older sister. She's always been adamantly opposed to marriage, even though she owns a home with her partner and they've been together for nine years. During my wedding, she was barraged with annoying, "When will it be your turn?" questions. And now, she's getting it again. Although Stacy has no intention of having a baby, people assume that since she is the older sister, she would be the first to have a baby. While I hope everyone will ask about my pregnancy, she's hoping for the opposite.

THE SHOWER IS OUT OF THE WAY, the birth supplies are standing at attention in the guest room, the labor tub is reserved, and I think I'm ready. The birth dream I have that night tells me I am.

I've had various pregnancy dreams, but this is my first birth dream. Everything in my abdomen starts moving toward my pelvic area. When I feel pressure against my pelvic floor muscles, I'm not afraid or in pain, only excited. When I wake, I realize the emotions are true. I'm no longer afraid of giving birth, even without medication. My prenatal yoga class, therapy sessions, and my body's insistent screams to "look at me!" have helped shift my perspective from being a failure at baby making to being a rock star. My girlie parts have succeeded for the past eight and a half months, I'm sure they'll do so when it comes time to deliver the baby. My body is in great shape. As long as I trust myself and don't let my brain start sliding back to a place of shame and fear, I think I'll do just fine. Everything is set.

Or so I thought, until my mom tells me she wants to be at the birth. It's not that I hadn't contemplated the idea myself, but once I rounded the bend to my last few weeks of pregnancy without her ever mentioning it, I assumed she didn't want to be there. I make the mistake of calling Stacy to commiserate. "Mom just told me she wants to be at the birth!"

"Yeah, I know. I want to be there too."

"What!? I'm thirty five weeks pregnant! Why are you guys only telling me this now?"

"I just assumed we'd be there. Didn't you?"

"No! I thought the whole thing freaked you out. I figured you'd come over once the birth stew was taken away and everything was cleaned up."

"Yeah, I'm not really into the messy parts, but I do want to be there."

Shit. I had it all worked out and really don't want a crowd. Especially a crowd that is unsure about home births (Stacy) or claims she blanks out in stressful situations, meaning the birth of her two daughters (my mom). They could be wonderful and helpful or they could be…. It's the unknown factor that makes me nervous. I don't want to hurt their feelings, yet after eight months of careful planning and mental preparation, I can't bear to throw a wild card into the mix. I need to feel in control of my birth environment and having a lot of people there feels out of control. I don't want anyone's fear and uncertainty spreading to me.

"I met a doula the other night at a party and she said…"

I can't help but interrupt Stacy. "Wait a minute, you know what a doula is? And you were actually socializing with one?"

"Yeah, you told me about them, remember?"

I remember explaining who Ellen was and why I wanted her at the birth, but I had assumed Stacy wasn't really paying attention.

"So this doula told me that it would be really helpful for you to have a lot of people at the birth. Maybe I won't jump in the birth stew with you, but I could make food and get you something to drink or run errands. She says there's always a lot to do and the more people the better."

"Interesting." I can't help but laugh at the absurdity of the conversation. Stacy quoting a doula, I never thought I'd see the day. "Let me think about it, OK?"

She's very convincing and what she says makes sense, but I still have my doubts. Better to talk to someone rational. Someone who isn't pregnant and who isn't related to Stacy. I look around the house for Jason.

I find him outside building a shed. He's been maniacal about this shed and various other house projects lately. Whenever I ask him what the rush is, he says, "I have to get this done before the baby is born!" Why a baby needs a storage shed, or new light fixture in the bathroom, I have no idea. But Jason seems to think it's of utmost importance.

As I watch him nervously reread the instructions, rub his chin, and then frantically hammer a few nails in, I wonder what happened to my calm and mellow husband. Who is this crazy person? I place my hand on his arm and ask him if he's all right. He nearly jumps out of his skin. "Shit, I didn't hear you coming. What are you doing?"

"Watching you."

"Why?"

"Because you seem a little tense. Are you OK?"

He tries to shrug off the question and mutters about the "stupid directions that are obviously missing a few pages or were translated by a monkey." When I probe a bit deeper, he admits that it's not just the shed he's worried about. He doesn't feel ready for the baby to come. "Up until our road trip, I thought I was ready. I read the books, attended most of the appointments with Afia, but now I'm not sure."

"Would it help to have Stacy or my mom here?"

He looks shocked. "I thought you only wanted Ellen, Lisa, and Afia here. Are you changing your mind?"

"No...well... I don't know. If you're getting nervous, maybe it would help you to have some back up as well. Then you wouldn't feel as if you have to do everything."

"That doesn't matter. You need to do what you want, what's going to make you comfortable."

I'm placing everyone else's needs before mine. I don't want to hurt anyone's feelings and I want Jason to have help, so I'm letting these things sway my own feelings. I take a second to close my eyes and ask myself what I want. The answer comes clearly and quickly.

"I want a quiet, unobtrusive birth with the people I've been working with."

"Then that's what we'll have." He smiles at me, but I still feel he's ill at ease. He knows I can see through his façade and says, "Don't worry about me, I'll be fine. I'll look over the books again, that will help."

"Is it the birth you're nervous about or becoming a father?"

"Both, I guess. I've been so fixated on you and the pregnancy and worried about another miscarriage that I realize I haven't done anything about me. You've made changes in your life, you quit your job, you're facing your past, but I haven't done any of that. One of the reasons I stalled you for so long was because I didn't want to be working at Ivey when we had a kid. I only got that job because Kevin worked there. It was never my dream to mount photos and advertisements all day long. I always thought I'd work there for a few months and then find something else. That I'd find something more interesting, more related to populations studies so I could feel as if I'm using my degree."

"But you tried to look for environmental jobs and saw they all involved working in an office, which you'd hate. You like working with your hands and being physical."

"I know, I guess that's why I've been at Ivey for ten years. I don't know what else to do. But I always thought I'd know by the time we had kids. I want to have a job that's interesting, that inspires me, not just something I fell into and haven't had the courage to leave. I want our child to be proud of me. For me to be able to say, 'You can be anything you want in this world,' and have our child believe me. But why would they, when I'm not doing what I want to do?"

"What do you want to do?"

"I don't know. That's the problem. And maybe it's too late. I can't give up my job and benefits, we have a baby coming."

"It's not too late. Maybe a new job would pay even better than your job now. Or if you want to go back to school, we could apply for financial aid. You're not stuck because of the baby, you're only stuck because you don't know what you want to do. But as soon as you do, I bet there are a lot of options."

"I hate the idea of having to start over. I'm the one people come to at Ivey with questions, and I like that. If I start over, I won't know anything."

"Maybe, but at least you won't be bored."

He doesn't look convinced. The "what should I be when I grow up?" question has plagued Jason off and on for years. I used to ask him a thousand and one questions about his interests, what kind of work setting he enjoys, and what his priorities are. Money, success, creativity, flexibility, camaraderie, working alone, or being in charge? But after years of playing career counselor, I realized it doesn't work to be a counselor and a wife, and I'd rather be his wife. Only he can decide what he wants to do with his life and I hope he decides soon. Otherwise he may blame me and the baby for feeling stuck.

"I was thinking about taking some time off once the baby is born to think about it. I still have a few weeks of vacation pay and you know Ryan, from work? He told me the Family Medical Leave Act allows you to take up to twelve weeks off without risking losing your job. He took ten weeks off when his son was born."

"I didn't know you could do that."

"I'll talk to the HR person this week. I don't know about taking three months off, but a month would be cool. We could afford that."

He looks at the ground and starts swinging his hammer back and forth. Unlike me, who processes out loud, Jason keeps most of his processing to himself.

"You could finish the shed then." I joke as a way to bring him back to me. I can see that he's drifted off and I want to know where he's gone.

"Are you worried about the birth?" I ask.

"A little. I mean, I know having it at home is the right choice and Afia seems to know what to do in any situation and we're only a few minutes from the hospital, but…. Well, you know how I am. I don't like winging it. I like to have a plan."

"We have a plan. I want to labor for as long as possible at home and hopefully birth the baby in the labor tub."

"Yeah, but what about me? What do you need from me?"

"I just need you to be you." That doesn't seem to help, so I continue with, "I need you to be present. To be with me. To be calm, supportive, and loving, that's all."

He nods his head.

"And if you don't feel calm, fake it. Or leave the room, OK?"

He laughs, but I can see he's still worried.

"Do you want to take a birthing class together? Would that help?"

"Yeah! Can we still get into one?" His face brightens for the first time since I've been outside. I see the creases ease around his eyes and am relieved to have some insight and a possible solution to some of what is worrying him. I leave him to his hammering and go inside to call Afia.

AFIA TELLS ME ABOUT a one-day crash course birthing class that may still have room. I call the birthing center and register immediately. I have been lukewarm about attending a birthing class, because, so far, it's been very healing to trust myself, rather than to elicit guidance from "experts." I hope my body will know what to do; and if it doesn't, Ellen and Afia will help me. But Jason loves directions and instructions. If it will help his confidence and alleviate stress for him, I'll happily sit through a birthing class.

Nina's birth experience showed me the value in people being able to intuit a laboring woman's needs. Nina was basically silent throughout her entire labor, but somehow her partner Tony was able to discern what she needed and how to help her. I want the same from Jason. I don't want to have to give directions or tell him what to do, nor do I want him to feel as if he has to instruct me. I just want him to be a calm, steady presence next to me.

When the alarm clock goes off in the morning, I groan. "Are you sure you really want to go to this class? How much can we really learn in four hours?"

"A lot. And we're going, so you better get up," Jason replies. He hops out of bed and goes downstairs to make coffee.

I complain all the way there, but start to feel a shift in attitude as I watch four very large women waddle into the birthing center. I thought I'd be the only procrastinator, but the other participants are thirty-five, thirty-six, even thirty-seven weeks along. At thirty-five weeks, I feel as if I've got plenty of time.

The main focus of the class is to help the birthing partner come up with various ways to assist the laboring woman. Equally stressed is what not to do—things that will result in the partner being screamed at or physically hurt. The class may only be four hours long, but it's packed with useful information. At the break, Jason chats with the other participants, makes jokes, and looks more at ease than I've seen him in weeks. By the end of class, he's walking with his head tall and his shoulders straight. "I think I got it," he says proudly.

"I know you do," I agree.

We head for the door, secure in our birth class knowledge, but stop when an ambulance pulls up and blocks our way. We ask our instructor what's going on and she says the woman in the room next to us is having some difficulties and the ambulance is here to help. She's trying to remain calm, but I can tell she's nervous. We knew a woman was laboring in the suite next to us, but we've hardly heard a peep out of her.

One of the midwives approaches us in the foyer, and calmly but urgently explains that it may be a little while before we can leave because the entrance needs to be free for the paramedics and fire truck. "Fire truck?" I ask, but no one hears me over the deafening sound of sirens. Within minutes, the room is overtaken by paramedics barking orders and yelling into walkie-talkies. The new age music, soft tinkling of a fountain in the corner, and the smell of lavender candles burning are all forgotten and in their place are stretchers, oxygen masks, defibrillators and very large, loud men.

Our instructor explains that the woman has been laboring for several hours without progressing. She's exhausted and is choosing to go to the hospital for pain relief. She and the baby aren't in danger; she just wants some relief so she can rest.

Although I've imagined transferring to the hospital many times, the image never included paramedics, sirens, or metal gurneys. Perhaps naively, I thought I would get in our car and Jason would drive me. The lights and sirens are jarring, and instead of feeling comforted by the sight of the paramedics, I feel tense. They don't belong in this setting of soft spoken women and dim lighting. I imagine them entering my own home and shudder.

I don't want to become too attached to any birth scenario, because that could be setting myself up for disappointment, but I also now know that having sirens and ambulances at my house will be traumatic. And once I'm inside the hospital, the bright lights and hustle and bustle aren't going to go away. I tell myself if I really need it, I'll be so relieved to see the paramedics or nurse, I won't care how noisy they are. But I'm not sure I believe myself.

THE NOTION OF COMFORT is taking on a whole new meaning. As I drive to friends' houses, I rack my memory for details of their furniture. Even though he can rarely answer the question, I ask Jason, "Does Chris have pregnant-friendly furniture?"

"Last time we were there, we sat on the floor. It was either that or that couch he found for free on the street."

"Ugh," I shudder. "That thing stinks. I wouldn't touch it without wearing a hazmat suit."

Sitting on chairs—or sitting in general—for long periods of time doesn't work for me. Most chairs and sofas allow the person sitting in them to recline, which is agony for a large pregnant woman. I can do it while constantly rearranging twelve pillows to prop up my legs and back, but who has time for that? Lying on the floor is so much easier. I grab a couple of pillows, prop them around me and lay on my side. It's the only way to be comfortable for more than ten minutes. Except for when it's time for bed, then lying down proves to be laborious and unpleasant.

I have to navigate around six or seven pillows, a heating pad, a CD player with earphones, the cat, and a trying-to-sleep Jason. The pillows serve as an attempt to create the ideal sleeping position. The heating pad provides comfort to my lower back. The CD player's earphones are strapped to my belly every night in my attempt to familiarize the baby with music that will lull it to sleep once it's out of utero. Someone told me this theory actually works, so I play various Eels CDs to my unborn baby every evening. The cat serves no purpose other than to keep me awake at night with her loud purring or incessant licking. As for the sleeping Jason, he serves as a pillow when he's asleep and stationary, which is usually not the case by the time I stumble my way into the bed.

I love to sleep and I like to do so for at least nine hours in a row. That no longer happens. I tell myself that soon enough the baby will be out of my belly and I'll be able to sleep comfortably again. Afia crushes that fantasy at our next appointment when she tells me, "Newborns like to eat every two hours or so."

"How do they do that?" I ask.

"You nurse them," she laughs.

"In my sleep?"

"If you can, you're very lucky. Most new moms wake up to nurse, because they want to make sure their baby is securely latched."

"But when do I get to sleep?"

"When the baby does."

The room becomes very small and I think I'm going to hyperventilate. Every two hours? She's got to be screwing with me. I'll never survive on that. I want to nurse my baby for a year, does that mean I don't get to sleep for twelve more months? What have I gotten myself into?

"Time for your examination. Strip from the bottom down and hop up on to the table."

This appointment couldn't get any worse. First of all, I can't "hop up" on to anything. Even if I could, I won't willingly hop up on to anything with stirrups. I was actually starting to believe I was going to make it through my entire pregnancy without a vaginal exam. Just like I thought I'd sleep all night with my baby. I'm so naïve.

No one actually likes gynecological exams, but I break out in a nervous sweat just thinking about them. I can't relax, or let my knees "fall open" as instructed, or stop from flinching as soon as I see the speculum. I've been this way since my first heinous exam where the doctor announced that sex would be very painful for me because I was "so tight." Maybe that was his version of teaching abstinence.

The botched biopsy, cervical freezing to cure the dysplasia, and rapes only increased my fear of the stirrups. I stare blankly at Afia and don't move.

"All right, we'll start slow. Let's feel your belly." She turns around to get her Doppler so we can hear the baby's heartbeat. I love hearing the baby and the thought of doing so alleviates some of my nervousness about the upcoming exam. I wiggle on to the table and let her palpate my belly. She giggles and says, "Hello there," as my baby moves towards her hands.

"You've got a lover in there. Every time I touch your belly, the baby scoots near my hands. I bet this will continue after the birth. The baby will be a real snuggler."

A Braxton Hicks contraction tightens across my abdomen, just as it always does these days when my belly is palpated. I try to relax and think about a snuggly baby lying next to me when Afia asks me to lay back. She props some pillows up on the examining table for me and helps me lean back into them. She places a skeleton of a woman's pelvis on my belly and shows me all of the areas she is going to measure in order to be confident that the baby's head and body can fit through my pelvis. Seems a little late to be determining that, but I listen anyway.

She hands me a velvet robe to drape over my legs and asks me if I'm ready to take my pants off. My palms begin to sweat at the idea. By now, I'm quite familiar with telling myself, "That was then, this is now." I remind myself that Afia is nothing like the other practitioners I've had and that I'm safe with her. I can tell her whenever it feels too much for me, and she'll stop. I am safe. I am safe.

She smiles at me and I nod. I slide my pants off and cover myself with the robe. So far, so good. I'm not sweating anymore, but I still feel uneasy. She turns the faucet on full blast to warm up the speculum, and pulls the stirrups out from the table. They are covered with sheepskin and look nothing like the stirrups from my past. *That was then, this is now.*

I feel uncharacteristically calm as I place my feet into the stirrups. I can't let my legs fall apart, so Afia talks to me some more. She explains what she's going to do and asks me to look at the pelvic skeleton while she talks. Focusing on the skeleton in combination with listening to Afia's nurturing voice alleviates some of my fear and I'm able to let my legs fall apart. I like knowing what Afia is going to do before she does it; it makes me feel in control. I also like being able to focus on something else besides the speculum inside of me.

Throughout the exam, she continues to talk to me. She explains where her hand is and what it's measuring and repeatedly checks in with me. And before I know it, it's over. I'm reassured that my pelvis is plenty wide, that my tailbone will not get in the way (I didn't even know that was a concern), and that the baby should have plenty of room for delivery.

I close my legs immediately, but don't get off the table. "Really?" I ask. "That's it?"

"Yeah," she laughs. "You can get dressed now."

That wasn't so bad, I think as I slide off the table. *And it's over. I won't have to have another one for at least a year.*

VI
Birth

Birth

I'M WORKING ESPECIALLY HARD on the December issue of *Women of Seattle*—maybe because it's the last issue of the year, or maybe because it's my last issue before I go on maternity leave. Either way, I want it to be a special issue. I'm surprised that I'm still motivated. My teaching skills are obviously suffering and the only thing I seem to get excited about these days is food, but somehow I'm still able to find pleasure in editing.

We start our production meeting with Karen telling us about how she and Faith spent the weekend working on the ever-evolving business plan. Faith interjects, "We should tell them the big news."

I feel my stomach tighten. The last "big news" resulted in me having a cut in my paycheck. Faith announces that they have decided not to print the December issue in order to save money. They rattle off all the benefits of this idea and the other ideas they have, but I can't focus on them. I can't believe they're canceling the issue after I already worked so hard on it. What am I going to tell the writers?

Several questions, and profanities, race through my mind as I try to explain to them calmly yet firmly that this is a bad idea. Karen and Faith nod, say it is a lot to consider, and we agree not to make a decision until we meet again next week.

I leave Faith's house relieved, but as soon as I get into my car, I'm concerned. Even if they print the December issue, the future of the paper doesn't look good. It's only a matter of time before it folds all together. I've been hoping that I'll be able to continue working for the paper while caring for my baby at home, but that probably won't happen.

I tell myself I don't know anything yet, so I shouldn't worry. Yes, I love my job and yes, I desperately want to be able to work from home, but so much of my fear is due to limited thinking. Maybe I can find an equally creative job. No matter what, I know I won't go back to a Fruitloop U situation. Now that I know what a difference having meaningful work can make, I'll try not to settle for less. It wouldn't be fair to me or my baby.

I know creative, flexible, fulfilling jobs are hard to find, but I also know if I found this one, I can find another one. It may take a while and it may not be perfect, but it is possible. And trying to sort out all of this now is futile. Although I've spent years trying, I can't control the future. I can prepare myself, work hard towards my desired outcome, but then I have to leave the rest up to fate. Just like I'm doing with my pregnancy.

My Zen thinking works for a while, but as soon as I get home, I start freaking out about not having a job. I tell myself I don't know this for sure yet and write "You don't need to have all of the answers now" on a piece of paper. I place it in the corner of the bathroom mirror along with "I am safe" and "I am good."

There's a lot I don't know and I need to accept that. My dubious editing career needs to take a backseat to the sure things in my life, which are: I am expected to teach for another week and my baby will be born within the month. That is plenty to focus on for now.

After teaching my last class, I ask the director of the school if I can check back with her in a few weeks to see what my future schedule will be. She laughs and says, "I don't expect to hear from you for a few months, but whenever you're ready, you know you can come back." I thank her and smile at her wisdom. There I go again, thinking I need to have all of the answers now.

I walk out of her office into the main office and tell the other teachers I'm off to deliver my baby. They laugh at me and say, "Yeah right, you still have another month to go." I'm almost thirty-eight weeks along, but the other teachers love seeing the look of horror on my face whenever they explain that first babies are always late.

But not my baby. My water breaks that night at five a.m. I knew my baby could hear me! I wake Jason up and call Afia. I describe the urinating sensation and color of the fluid, which assures Afia that my labor has started. She suggests we go back to sleep and rest as much as possible. Sleep! No way, I'm too excited. I ask Jason what he wants to do, but he doesn't answer. He's sound asleep and snoring softly.

I take a shower and get dressed, careful not to wake Jason. I return books to the library, buy some snacks and champagne at the grocery store, and even buy myself a decaf mocha. All the while, I think to myself, "I'm in labor right now and no one knows it. What a trip!" I get back to the house and make myself scrambled eggs, toast, a fruit smoothie, and slice up several grapefruits as well. There's still no sign of Jason, but I'm no longer careful to be quiet. I bang the pots and pans around while cleaning them and stomp up and down the stairs a few times until he wakes up.

I can feel the contractions, but they aren't debilitating, so Jason and I discuss what we want to do. "Looks like we're not going to get the pregnancy photos I wanted," I say. We have a photo shoot scheduled with my friend Lori this weekend, but we should have scheduled one sooner. I know Lori is working, so I can't call her now, but I could call Stacy. She's a good photographer and has a flexible schedule. Plus, I'm still feeling guilty about not letting her come to the birth. She and my mom both seemed fine about my decision, but I can't help feeling sorry that I may have hurt their feelings. I know Stacy wants to feel as if she is supporting me, so a nice compromise could be to have her take some photos for us. Jason says it's a good idea and I call Stacy.

She comes right over with her camera in hand and at least four rolls of film. We go upstairs to our bedroom where the morning light is best. It's a beautiful, sunny day, so we sit near the window where the sun pours over Jason and I. After taking a roll of pictures of Jason and me, Stacy suggests we move on to just me. We're going to take several close-ups of my belly, so I take my clothes off.

Ever since the girls at the salt water pool, I've been walking around naked as much as possible. And when I pass a mirror, I make myself stop and observe my body. I hope to capture the ease and comfort I felt at times in these photos. I know there may be a time when I feel insecure again, maybe as soon as when this baby is outside of me. But I hope these photos will remind me of a time when I felt confident. Maybe they'll even help me feel that way again.

After two hours of belly shots, full body nudes, and many tender poses with Jason, I feel confident that we have thoroughly documented my body and my pregnancy. I'm tired from the photo shoot and concerned that the contractions haven't strengthened. Jason remembers that long walks can progress a labor, so I get my clothes and shoes on. When Stacy claims she'll stay at our house and wait for us, Jason and I look at one another nervously.

"No, it's time for me to focus and be alone with Jason," I say. She puts up a bit of a fight, but eventually agrees to leave. She says, "I'm only a phone call away. I can be here in three minutes," as we walk her to the door.

We're just about to leave when the phone rings. It's Faith and she has a "little favor" to ask me. She wants to know if I will send her all of the December articles and email all of the writers to tell them that, although we are not going to print a December issue, we will place their articles on the paper's website.

"Faith," I explain, "maybe you didn't hear me. I'm in labor."

"I know, it's so exciting! This won't take long."

I grumble to myself, tell Jason I'll be ready in about an hour, and turn on my computer. The contractions increase in intensity as I work, but still don't feel like the "real thing." I can breathe my way through them and return to work relatively easily. As soon as they pass, I feel fine.

I email all of the writers and tell them if they have any concerns, they should contact Karen or Faith, because I'm busy having a baby. Once that's out of the way, we finally go for our walk. It's no longer sunny. It actually looks and feels as if it might rain. When we're about a mile and a half away from our house, the wind picks up and it starts to pour down rain. No gentle sprinkles as a warning, just a deluge. Running is no longer an option for me, so we walk as quickly as possible back home.

Although our walk is cut short, it does the trick by speeding up my labor. By the time we get home, I'm no longer able to talk during contractions. I'm tired, but lying down is extremely uncomfortable, so I walk around the house. It's around five in the afternoon and I'm feeling the effects of being awake for twelve hours. Damn it, I should have listened to Afia and slept when Jason did.

Jason calls Afia and after listening to me breathe and groan over the phone, she says she and her assistant will be there within the hour. She also suggests that I eat something. While Jason makes me a turkey sandwich, I walk and sway around the kitchen. When a contraction comes, I grab the kitchen counter, put my head down, squat, and moan. Movement seems to help, so although I would love to curl up in my bed and sleep, I keep moving.

Jason puts on a Woody Allen movie, remembering the suggestion from our birthing class that a movie can distract the laboring woman, but I can't stand still long enough to watch. We go upstairs and start walking in circles. He follows me through our room, the guest room, and back through our room. I've never appreciated our open floor plan more. Every time a contraction hits, I grab his hands and crouch down.

The pain increases in intensity and I say I need Ellen's help. The contractions are more debilitating and frequent and I'm getting nervous. Ellen tells Jason she'll be at our house in an hour or so, but he has the good sense to tell me she's on her way. An hour will sound like forever to me and I'll panic, but in actuality, I have no sense of time. Better to lie to me and hope I don't notice.

He calls the labor tub women next and asks them to bring the tub. They had instructed us to not call them until I was in active labor, because they know that first time labors can take a long time and the tub only stays warm for so long. He's not sure if I'm in "active" labor, but based on my groans, he sure hopes so. With all of the calls made, we walk and squat while we wait for our support team to arrive.

JASON AND I CIRCLE around our bed, through the two French doors to the guest room, around the stairs, and back through our room over a hundred times while we wait for Ellen to show up. But just as Jason hopes, I have no idea whether he called her five minutes or an hour ago.

Jason's hands lose all feeling and his arms are shaking from supporting my weight, so I adopt other things to hold on to. Jason's dresser is the perfect height for me to lean against and is heavy enough for me to be able to put all of my weight against it without it falling over. Plus, above it are two pictures that Jason took on our honeymoon in Ireland. It comforts me to look at all that lush greenery and remember a time when I wasn't in pain. The other stations are the ledge by our staircase and the wall separating Jason's closet from mine. I use all three places to lean, grunt, and breathe my way through the contractions while Jason strokes my back.

I'm holding on to the ledge and crouching when Ellen arrives. She immediately presses her hands against my sacrum while I sink into her hands. She's incredibly strong and knows exactly where to apply the pressure to relieve the tension of the contractions. She shows Jason how to do it and goes downstairs to get me something to drink and an ice pack. During each contraction, one of them holds the ice pack to my sacrum and one of them squeezes my hips. Both actions relieve the pressure I feel building in my lower back.

The labor tub woman arrives, unfolds the tub and fills it with hot water. The walls are about three and a half feet high and the tub is six feet in diameter. On top of the walls is a foam pad, for comfort. After two rounds from our hot water heater, the woman places the heater in the tub, covers it, and wishes me luck. Every time I pass by the tub, I look at it longingly. I'm not allowed to get in until Afia checks me. Since my water broke already, there's a potential for infection if I spend too much time in the water before I deliver the baby.

Shortly after the tub is set up, Afia and her assistant Lisa arrive. Once they set up their equipment, Afia says it's time to check me. I ignore her the first few times because I'm too entranced by what's going on inside my body to notice or hear anything else. Plus, I thought the exam I had in her office was the last one I'd have to have in a while so I don't understand what she's asking of me. It takes Afia and Jason walking me over to the bed, lying me down, and asking me to take my pants off for me to finally get it. Lying down hurts, and having her hand placed inside me is excruciating. Hearing I'm only one centimeter dilated and eighty percent effaced only increases my agony. Afia tells me not to worry about how far along I am and to continue to focus on one contraction at a time.

Jason and Ellen continue to follow me as I walk, sway, and moan. One of them continues to press the ice pack on my lower back or squeeze my hips and the other one holds my hands and breathes and sways with me. Although I'm in my own world and oblivious to my surroundings, gazing into one of their faces during the contractions helps me feel safe. I'm not alone, loved ones are near, and they are going to do everything they can to help me through this.

Whenever I stop moving, Afia's assistant Lisa crawls under me to check the fetal heart-rate with her Doppler. Afia sees that I'm in good hands, and goes downstairs to sleep. I could be in labor all night long and this may be her only chance to rest. I whimper with exhaustion every time we walk by our bed, futon, or the labor tub. It's after nine p.m. and I'm only one centimeter dilated. I'm tired and disappointed I'm not further along, but can barely think about it because I'm too busy concentrating on how to get through each contraction.

I remember my rocks and ask Jason for them. He places my rose quartz in my left hand and my river rock in the right. They fit perfectly in my hands and the weight of them is grounding. I run my fingers over their smoothness. And once a contraction hits, I squeeze the hell out of them. I know they can take any amount of squeezing and that's comforting. No matter what, they will stay with me.

By eleven p.m. the contractions are every two minutes and intense. I lay my head in Jason's lap after a contraction, fall asleep, dream, and then feel the baby kick and stand straight up. The baby always kicks before the contraction as a signal to get ready. If I don't stand and sway before the contraction peaks, it hurts even more.

My body is so tired that my legs start to shake. Ellen has me sit backwards on the toilet, but that proves to be very uncomfortable. We try several positions on my hands and knees as well, but I immediately go back to what feels right.

My body wants to stand and sway, so that's what I do. I'm shaking and having a hard time regulating my temperature, but my recent exam proves that it's still too soon to get in the tub. Although my cervix is difficult to find, Afia thinks I'm still only one centimeter dilated.

Shortly after the exam, the pain becomes much more intense. For the first time, "Can I do this?" goes through my mind. I'm completely nonverbal, and have been ignoring everyone in the room for hours, but Ellen senses my pain and fear and begins a new breathing technique with me. She holds my face in her hands and makes me hold eye contact with her by saying, "Look at me, Corbin, look at me." Once our eyes meet, she counts, "One, two, three, blow." Anytime I look away, she grabs my face and makes me look at her. We do this over and over again and my doubts disappear.

During a "One, two, three, blow" routine, Afia notices that my moans become grunts and can tell that I'm further along than she thought. She thinks I'm in transition and finally lets me get into the labor tub.

One foot into the tub and I'm a new person. My shivering stops and I feel warm, yet not too warm, for the first time all evening. Submerging in the water not only regulates my body temperature, it also eases my tired aching body. Jason holds me under my armpits and I let my legs stretch out in the water in between each contraction. When the contractions hit, I crouch, grab Ellen's hand, and stare at her through our "one, two, three, blow" routine. I absolutely have to do this every time otherwise I scream in agony and start to fear I won't make it. Ellen encourages me to take shallow breaths, almost like panting, but I scream, "No! I like the blows." She doesn't try to alter my breathing again.

I finally make it through transition and feel the desire to push. I didn't understand I was in transition. I just thought I was in hell and that the hell was going to get worse, but I understand that pushing means I'm near the end. Although it hurts a lot, it's a relief to feel as if I'm doing something to help my baby along rather than merely enduring the pain. Now I can work with the contractions instead of hoping they'll end soon.

"This is going to be the one. After this push, your baby's head will be out," Afia cheers several times, but she's wrong. The baby's head continues to slip back into my vagina. She tells me to put my hand down and feel my baby's head, but I don't hear her. I'm too focused on coping with the "train running over me while trying to push a watermelon out" feeling. When she mentions it a third time, I release my death grip from Jason's arm and feel between my legs. "It's squishy!" I squeal. What a relief to feel it so close. If I could only get it to stay out.

Afia places a mirror on the bottom of the labor tub so I can watch the baby's head crown with every push. I glance at it a few times, but mostly I focus on Jason's or Ellen's face as I squeeze their hands and scream. Afia keeps warning me that all my screaming will make me hurt tomorrow, but I couldn't care less. There's no way a sore throat will hurt more than delivering this baby.

After two hours of pushing and twenty-one hours of labor, the head and the elbow nestled next to the head finally emerge. A few pushes later, the shoulders and body come out and the baby is placed on my belly. Jason and Ellen burst into tears, but all I feel is relief. I have a huge grin on my face. I look at my baby and say, "Thank God you're here. Thank God that's over."

The baby and I relax in the warm water while Afia and Lisa check our vitals. Lisa places a hat on the baby and takes my blood pressure. At least ten minutes pass before I ask what the sex is. Afia laughs, "I don't know, take a look." I raise the baby up and say, "It's a boy!"

Although I started to think I was having a girl, my whole body relaxes at the knowledge that I have a boy. My sexual trauma makes me uncertain of how I would raise a girl. I'd want her to be strong, to honor her sexuality, and to not be afraid, yet all of these attributes are so muddy for me. How would I teach a girl to be sexual and not be afraid of men, given my own experience of being raped?

Holding this beautiful boy in my arms feels so right and simple in comparison. I know I'll instill in him a respect for women. And knowing he'll have Jason as a gentle role model allows me to feel fairly confident that our baby will grow up to be a compassionate, respectful adolescent.

My daydreams about raising a kindhearted, considerate boy are interrupted when Jason asks, "Why is there a red towel in the tub?"

It's not a towel, it's blood. I'm hemorrhaging.

MY UTERUS DOESN'T CONTRACT after I deliver the placenta so I continue to bleed. A lot. Lisa roughly massages my uterus in hopes that it will start to contract on its own. When that doesn't work, Afia administers an intra-muscular injection to my leg in order to stop the bleeding. The bleeding slows, but is still alarming. Afia guides me to my bed, rolls up her sleeves, and says, "I'm sorry, you're not going to like this one bit, but I have to do it." I know exactly what she's going to do, based on Lydia's birth, and brace myself for the pain. Afia bodyslams herself down on my uterus until the bleeding slows down.

Once she is certain that I'm no longer hemorrhaging, Afia addresses my poor perineum. "Wow, he really did a number on you. His head is extremely large, but it was that elbow that really did the damage. It's as if it dug a trench right through you." Jason joins Afia at the foot of the bed to see what she is talking about. "Yikes," he says and goes back to singing and pacing with our baby. Afia warns me that administering the Novocain and the actual stitching of my perineum might be uncomfortable, but I don't feel a thing. I'm too elated. Not only am I able to lie on my back comfortably for the first time in months, but I have a baby! The labor is finally over! I did it!

I look around the room, having been completely unaware of my surroundings for hours, and notice Lisa putting the medical equipment that covers most of my bedroom floor away. "Holy crap! What is all of that stuff?" I ask.

"Oxygen for the baby, adult oxygen mask, ambu bag for neonatal resuscitation, herbs, homeopathics, anti-hemorrhagic medications, IV fluids, magnesium sulphate for high blood pressure, epenephrine for anaphalactic shock due to antibiotic sensitivity, IV antibiotics, injectable Vitamin K and erythromycin eye prophylactic for newborn, baby scale, blood pressure cuff, stethoscope, hand held Doppler, umbilical clamps, butterfly needles, tourniquet...." I don't understand half of what Lisa's saying, but laugh at the myth that a homebirth only involves boiling water and getting towels ready.

Once Afia finishes with the stitches, I prop myself up in bed and hold my arms out for the baby. I'm still naked and the baby immediately finds my nipple. As he nurses away, I grin like an idiot. Ellen brings up five plates of left-over cannelloni and we dig in. Once all of the food is eaten, Ellen asks if we have a name for the baby. Jason and I shake our heads in unison. We couldn't decide on a name without first meeting and getting to know our baby. The name will be with him his whole life; I feel no need to make a rash choice.

The sun comes up and I see it's six in the morning. Twenty five hours without sleep is taking its toll. The women intuit this, and after cleaning the house and tucking us into bed, they leave. Jason and the baby fall right asleep, but I can't. I look around the room and can't believe a birth just occurred. Everything looks so normal and calm. Music is playing softly, the smell from extinguished aromatherapy candles still fills the air, and the furniture is back in place. It feels like any other day, except for the cooing baby in my arms.

I'm so relieved to have the experience behind me. No more discussing all of Jason's backwoods emergency procedures or worrying about something going wrong. I bet he is secretly disappointed that he didn't get to use any of the emergency techniques he had so carefully studied.

Even hemorrhaging, one of the things I feared the most, wasn't a crisis. Afia's voice became sharp in her directions to Lisa, but besides that, it seemed as if everything was under control, and no one panicked. My mind never raced to, "I better get to the hospital," nor did I doubt that Afia couldn't handle it. I just listened to her advice, prepared my body for the body slams, and then it was over.

Transferring to a hospital never entered my mind. Thanks to the diligence of Ellen and Jason, I was able to stay focused and cope with the contractions. Even when I entered transition, the farthest my mind went was, "God, this hurts!" I never thought about drugs because Ellen's breathing technique kept me focused and helped me forget about the pain. Yes, there was an enormous amount of pain, but I was able to view it as work, not as debilitating. And Afia was right, the work paid off and it gave me the thing I've been dreaming about for years. A baby.

Jason was supportive and calm and knew when to talk and when to be quiet, without me ever having to guide him. He pushed on my back when I needed it and was always within arm's reach. And when I needed it most, he provided a secure, comfortable lap for me to sleep on between contractions.

I never felt uneasy about my past sexual traumas or uncomfortable being stark naked and screaming in front of Ellen, Lisa, Jason, Afia or the labor tub woman for that matter. My only concern was making it through each contraction. Although I didn't research or read a lot of books, my body found its own rhythm and coping mechanisms. It knew what it needed and I listened to it.

I don't remember ever feeling frightened, insecure, or as if I wanted to give up. At one point, without thinking about it, I began chanting, "I can do this, I can do this," over and over again. My horoscope from eight months ago was right. I climbed the mountaintop, gained perspective on my life, and then focused solely on my most important goal—having a baby. My mental, emotional, and physical "training" paid off and I was able to birth a healthy baby at home. When I needed help, I listened to Ellen. When I felt confident in what I was doing, I ignored the other's advice and followed my own.

Now, if I can just remember this and employ it in my every day life.

VII
Epilogue

Epilogue

I SPEND THE DAYS in awe of my baby. We leave the house once a day to go for a short walk, but besides that, all I do is stare at him. Visitors come and go and shower us with attention and gifts. They almost always find us curled up on the living room couch, grinning like fools.

Afia is right, damn her, and my baby wants to nurse every hour or two. I quickly lose function of my brain, start babbling incoherently, and bump into walls. It reminds me of being pregnant. After a few weeks of this, I start to wonder if I'll ever feel intelligent again.

I miss working, but am not sure I'm mentally or physically capable yet. I sit in my rocking chair and ask my nursing baby, "What should I do?" I don't think he knows. Why should he? He's not even a month old. He doesn't even have a name yet. I know he's bright, but that's for me to figure out, not him.

I check in with Faith and Karen and they fill me in on their plan to raise capital for the paper. Some funds are gathered, the paper's look and feel is changed again, but within a few months, it ceases being published, this time for good.

I call the director I most recently taught for and she tells me I can bring my baby to work with me. I agree to teach again on a part time basis. I spend the rest of my time trying to sleep or write. I jot ideas and stories down in notebooks, on napkins, and on diapers. Every once in a while, I actually type some of these stories onto my laptop. I'm not sure what I'll do with them, but it feels good to be using my brain for something creative again.

When Conor is four months old—yes, it took a month, but we finally settle on a name—Jason uses his vacation time to take a month long leave of absence from his job. He researches an environmental certificate program and decides to enroll. The certificate takes nine months to complete and the classes are held in the evening. It's a nice compromise—being able to take a step towards making a change in his life without quitting his job.

Afia's prediction that we'd have a snuggler turns out to be true. Conor spends the majority of his time in my arms. The only time he's not happy is when I dare to put him down. Although this is endearing, my shoulders are screaming in agony and sometimes I really want the use of all of my limbs. During Jason's time off from work, I bask in having another person around to hold Conor.

We head to the coast for a few weeks to celebrate our new family. While there, Jason is able to give me lots of breaks by taking Conor for walks and drives. When they're gone, I try to clear the fog from my head and write. I type incoherent ramblings into my computer. The ramblings become jumbled essays and, put together, the essays sort of resemble a book. An idea is formed.

"This is supposed to be a vacation," Jason teases one day. "Why are you spending so much time on the computer?"

"It's a luxury to write. When I'm at home, I don't have any time, but while you take care of Conor, I can focus."

"What are you working on?"

"Breaking the silence."

"Huh?"

"I want to write a book about us and the rape and why I chose to birth Conor at home."

"Isn't that personal? Are you sure you want everyone to know all that stuff?"

"For now, I'm just writing it for myself. To get it all out and stop pretending it doesn't exist. But eventually, I think I'll be ready to share it with other people."

"Really? Wouldn't you be scared?"

"If I'm scared, I'm not ready," I say. "But I think some day sharing this story in a big way will feel right. I know it would help me to feel as if I'm not keeping a secret anymore and maybe some other women with similar situations will relate as well. I'll know when the time is right to share it." I pause, then add, "And until then, I'll write it for myself."

Acknowledgements

I would like to thank Waverly, Courtney, and Emily for calling me a writer before I believed that about myself. And to my writer's group, for boosting me up and slowing me down, I love you all. My eternal gratitude to Mike and Nancy for their unwavering support and especially for the use of their beautiful Tree House. Being there almost made the seemingly endless task of revising this book bearable.

Jess, you appeared as the New Year's gift I'd been dreaming about for years and your enthusiasm and encouragement has never waned. I couldn't ask for a better editor, thank you. To Jason, for always allowing me to write what I need to write, even when it's about you. None of this would have been possible without my midwives in life. Lisa, Eileen, Macky, Afia, Jennifer, Diane, Marcie, Jill, Diana, Erika, Courtney, Marcia, Lori and Deb continue to encourage me to fly and are always there to pick up the pieces when I fall. Thank you. My life is so much richer with you in it.

And finally, but certainly not least, to Conor and Stella who make my heart soar every day. Thank you for understanding why I need to shut myself in the purple room and bang on those white keys for hours on end. You are my inspiration, my teachers, often my muse. I couldn't be more honored and proud to have you in my life.

Corbin Lewars
Seattle, Washington, June 2009

Catalyst Book Press

Available Now

Are you Famous? Touring America with Alaska's Fiddling Poet
by Ken Waldman

Ken Waldman has toured throughout North America as Alaska's Fiddling Poet since 1995. He is the author of six poetry collections and has released seven CDs. This, his first book of prose, is part memoir, part travel notes, and part artist how-to. A *Blue Highways* for 2009. "A suggested must-read for our staff." —Scott D. Stoner, Chief Program Officer, Association of Performing Arts Presenters, Washington D.C.

Now also available with Ken's latestCD
Some Favorites-20 Tunes, 11 Poems, Surprises

Labor Pains and Birth Stories:
Essays on Pregnancy, Childbirth, and Becoming a Parent
essays edited by Jessica Powers, intro by Tina Cassidy

Giving birth is a time when one's best dreams and ideas—and worst fears and nightmares—coalesce into a single moment of anticipation. Out of such moments are birthed stories that reach into the deepest place of what it means to be human, what it means to be a spiritual being, what it means to love and be loved. "Where oh where was *Labor Pains and Birth Stories* when I was pregnant? By turns hilarous and heartbreaking, this book is destined to become a baby shower must-give." —Jennifer Niesslein, co-founder of *Brain, Child: The Magazine for Thinking Mothers* and author of *Practically Perfect in Every Way.*

LaVergne, TN USA
19 September 2010
197610LV00005B/24/P